£1 -20

GW00320281

# Dr Mike Smith's
# Handbook of Over-The-Counter Medicines

DR MIKE SMITH in an NHS Consultant in Public Health Medicine and President of the Association of Broadcasting Doctors. He was the Chief Medical Officer of the Family Planning Association 1970–75 and their Honorary Medical Adviser 1975–90. He is also a founder member of the National Food Safety Advisory Centre Expert Panel.

He has been an expert guest on the *Jimmy Young Programme* once a fortnight for 15 years; an expert guest on LBC once a week for ten years; and the medical columnist/editor on *Woman's Own* for 15 years. Between 1980 and 1984 he presented BBC1's health series *Looking Good, Feeling Fit*, and from 1988–90 he was an expert guest on SKY TV's *Weekly Magazine*. In April 1991 he was voted the TV and Radio Doctors' 'Expert's Expert' in the *Observer* magazine's series.

His other books include *Birth Control, How to Save Your Child's Life* and *A New Dictionary of Symptoms*.

# Dr Mike Smith's Handbook of Over-The-Counter Medicines

KYLE CATHIE LIMITED

First published in Great Britain in 1992 by
Kyle Cathie Limited
3 Vincent Square London SW1P 2LX

ISBN 1 85626 049 6

A CIP catalogue record for this book is available from the British
Library.

Designed by Beverley Waldron
Edited by Caroline Taggart
Typeset by DP Photosetting, Aylesbury, Bucks
Printed and bound in Great Britain by
Butler & Tanner Ltd, Frome and London

# Contents

# Acknowledgements

For her extensive research on this book, a thousand thanks go to journalist Sharron Kerr, my colleague and friend.

My thanks also go to Joan Tillott MRPhS and Nazleen Meghji MRPhS of Tillott and Tongue District Pharmacy – my local chemists – and to the pharmaceutical companies who readily sent details of their products.

# Foreword –
# How to Use this Book

THIS BOOK IS divided into two main sections. The first is an A-Z of common complaints, describing the symptoms and the 'self-help' measures you can take to treat them. At the end of each entry, there is a list of remedies, including homoeopathic and herbal remedies, available over the counter and suitable for the treatment of the complaint. The second section is an alphabetical list of the remedies themselves, giving details of the active ingredients and dosages recommended. A third, shorter section discusses vitamins, minerals and other supplements you may want or need to add to your diet.

All the medicines listed in both sections continue to sell and be recommended by doctors and pharmacists. They have all proved themselves reliable in their own ways. But the cause of many of the conditions they are taken to relieve is unknown – cramp in a young, fit person, for example. The fact that one remedy will work for one person and that another will suit someone else better may be because, for many conditions, there is more than one cause. So it's only to be expected that there should be more than one effective remedy. A certain amount of trial and error may sometimes be required before you find the remedy that is right for you or your child.

However, to guide you further, I have whenever possible suggested my favourite or favourites among the remedies available for each complaint. I do this just because they *are* my favourites and are popular – they are the ones I will most often recommend for patients or choose for myself or my family. Although they are my first choice, the other remedies given may be equally effective in their own way for some people.

Also, time passes and medicines come and go. Just because a medicine isn't mentioned here, it doesn't mean it isn't effective and doesn't have a role. And although I've tried to be comprehensive, it is inevitable – simply because of the numbers involved – that some medicines will have been overlooked. However, if you let me know, care of the publishers, about any of your favourite medicines I've missed, I'll do my best to include them in the next reprint of the book.

Other doctors and pharmacists will have their own favourites. When these differ from mine, I hope you'll forgive me and that you will take their advice first, since they have the privilege of being able to talk to you personally and assess your individual symptoms.

Their advice should also be sought about the quality and price (usually cheaper) of 'own brand' drugs – those common medicines like soluble aspirin produced for the local chemist to sell 'under their own label', rather than the nationally known and advertised 'brand' products like Disprin.

# Introduction

IN A DEVELOPED country like Britain most of the conditions the majority of us suffer from are self-limiting – they get better on their own. Among the common ones are colds, flu, gastric upsets, coughs, aches, strains, sprains, sore throats – even verrucas. While rest, possibly in bed, relaxes the body and keeps the patient at an even temperature, it's the body's own defences which deal with the infection or inflammation – the cause of almost all the conditions or their symptoms.

But even though most of us realise that it's just a matter of time before we recover from the nastiest cold or stomach upset, few can resist the temptation to try and hurry the process along or to relieve the pain or distress of the symptoms. So we treat ourselves with the tried and trusted remedies that have been used for generations and can be bought 'over the counter' (OTC). And powerful 'cures' many of them are, too. They often rely on the best of the plant-derived remedies of old. Aspirin, for example, which came originally from the bark of a certain type of willow tree, remains one of the best all purpose painkillers, temperature-reducing agents and anti-inflammatory agents available.

Some over-the-counter medicines can be bought in a supermarket, but all of them are available at the chemist's – the shop with the big difference where medicines are concerned. There, all medicines are kept or overseen by a professional pharmacist. He or she knows about and can advise on any of the medicines that are sold – or dispensed, when you hand in a doctor's prescription.

Fortunately, we are all getting healthier in Britain, so with every year that passes the pharmacist's role becomes more important. It is to the pharmacist that we should turn for everyday medical queries – as, in a way, we have done for centuries. The drug-dispensing apothecary of old was the forebear of both the modern-day family doctor and the pharmacist. While the family doctor specialises in diagnosis and takes overall professional responsibility for the care of our more serious illnesses, the pharmacist has the direct care and control of the medicines we take on a day-to-day basis.

**Making the Most of your Pharmacist**  A pharmacist's training involves three or four years of study, followed by a year's practical work under supervision. After this, their knowledge of the way drugs act upon the body and interact with each other – and the potential side-effects of them all – is considerable. Community pharmacists – the official name for retail pharmacists or chemists – are therefore highly qualified professionals. They are also available throughout shop opening hours, so your local pharmacist is probably the most accessible member of the healthcare team to whom you can go for free advice. Unfortunately, not many of us take full advantage of their expertise.

Most simple ailments don't need a prescription medicine. So if you don't feel well but don't think it's worth bothering your doctor, go to your local chemist and ask if you can speak to the pharmacist. He or she is trained to know when medical help is necessary, so if you are advised to go to the doctor, do so. Often, however, reassurance and an over-the-counter remedy will be all you need – and this guide is designed to help you understand the wide range of over-the-counter remedies available.

But there are certain basic precautions you must always take. Make sure you tell the pharmacist if you are already taking any medicines and if you are sensitive to anything. If you are asking advice about a child, always mention their age. If the pharmacist sells you some medicine, make sure you know how it should be taken and for how long, and follow the instructions precisely. Never exceed the recommended dose, unless it's on medical advice.

It's also worth mentioning here that the pharmacist and doctor act as a team when dealing with prescription medicines. It's part of the pharmacist's job to check that details on the prescription are correct before supplying it, make sure medicines are labelled properly and instructions fully understood. People are often nervous when they consult their doctor and may therefore not be quite clear about the treatment prescribed. They may also forget to mention any non-prescription medicines they are taking. You can always ask your pharmacist about anything you do not understand and check, if necessary, that your medicines will not react badly together. If you notice symptoms that you think may be due to a medicine's side-effects, the pharmacist will be able to tell you whether or not this is likely and advise you accordingly.

Pharmacists can also give advice on such things as immunisations for holidays abroad, headaches, stomach upsets, colds and coughs. They know, for instance, that different types of cough require quite different medicines, and will make sure you buy the right thing. Indeed, many of the more effective non-prescription medicines can only be supplied under the supervision of a pharmacist, so you need have no fear of being advised by someone who doesn't know what they're doing.

Certain medicines can be supplied either on prescription or over-the-counter. The over-the-counter price is sometimes cheaper than the prescription charge and it is worth asking your pharmacist's advice on this. New regulations mean that medicines are now often dispensed with information leaflets which include details of any side-effects that may occur. This knowledge could mean that more people expect to experience side-effects and therefore do so. In this case, the pharmacist is just the person to give advice or reassurance.

Many chemist shops now have a quiet area where you can talk to the pharmacist privately. On-the-spot pregnancy tests, blood-pressure checks and more recently, checks for cholesterol (blood fat) levels and general health and dietary advice are often available.

Most people will find it helpful to get to know their local pharmacist and build up a good relationship. To young mothers and the elderly in particular, a friendly pharmacist can be a valuable source of knowledgeable advice and support.

**Homoeopathy**   No one has so far been able to explain why homoeopathy works, as it does not conform to our accepted knowledge of scientific medicine. This method of giving medicines was first developed nearly 200 years ago by Dr Samuel Hahnemann, a great German physician, scholar and chemist. Appalled by the existing medical practices which he believed often did more harm than good, he sought a method of treatment which would be safe, gentle and effective. Since then many thousands of people throughout the world have had their symptoms relieved thanks to homoeopathy and even the Queen is said to carry a 'first-aid kit' of homoeopathic remedies with her on her travels. Homoeopathic medicines are widely recognised as a safe and effective alternative to conventional medicines.

Derived from the Greek word *homoios*, meaning 'like', homoeopathy's basic principle is that like cures like. Symptoms are treated by giving a minute dose of a substance which, if given in larger quantities to a healthy person, would actually cause those symptoms. Even in conventional medicine this principle is sometimes used – for instance, controlled doses of radiation are given to cure cancer which can be caused by too much radiation.

Over the years 'provings' have been carried out on many hundreds of substances by giving minute doses to healthy people and carefully noting the symptoms produced. Homoeopathic remedies are now based on these provings. The success of the treatment largely depends, homoeopaths say, on correctly matching the remedy to the individual's symptoms; other factors such as the patient's personality, home environment and work, which may have a bearing on the illness, can also play an important role in the choice of treatment. There are around 2,000 homeopathic remedies, each with several uses, so it is fortunate that computers can now be used to help in the matching-up process.

Visiting a homoeopath can be a lengthy business. He or she needs to build up a picture not only of your illness, but also of your personality and lifestyle, down to the tiniest detail of your favourite foods and even your reaction to weather! Homoeopaths believe that symptoms – for example, a raised temperature, running nose, diarrhoea or vomiting – are the body's way of trying to rid itself of whatever is responsible for the illness. They also believe in the body's natural ability to heal itself. A homoeopath will therefore aim to give a remedy which will encourage this process, whereas conventional doctors prescribe medicines to suppress symptoms – aspirin, for instance, is used to bring down a temperature, or antihistamines to dry up a runny nose.

Some homoeopathic remedies are similar to herbal medicines in that they are derived from plants, but many come from minerals such as gold, carbon, silica (sand) and phosphorus, or animal products such as bee stings or snake venom. Another class of remedies, called nosodes, are derived from disease tissue, bacteria or viruses, and are used as a form of vaccination against allergies and some illnesses or inherited conditions.

The methods of preparing homoeopathic remedies and dosages are quite different to those used in herbal medicine (see below). In homoeopathy, different 'potencies' of medicine are achieved by diluting, to varying degrees, a 'mother tincture' made from the initial substance. At each stage of dilution the mixture is thoroughly shaken – a process known as succussion.

'Less is more' is another basic principle of homoeopathy. In other words, contrary to what one might expect, the more dilute the solution, the more powerful its action will be. Medicines are graded according to this potency. The greater the dilution, the higher the potency number given to the remedy. So, for example, a homoeopathic remedy labelled 12c, which has been diluted 1,200 times, is of a lower potency than one labelled 30c, which has been diluted 3,000 times. 200c is a higher potency still.

The bottle or tube of medicine will have a number indicating its strength. Over-the-counter preparations will probably be 6c or the stronger 30c, though homoeopaths may prescribe higher. Homoeopaths find that high potencies – when only one dose is necessary – are better for some conditions and lower potencies, perhaps used for longer, better for others. Any potency above 12c will be so diluted that no particle of the original material can be found on chemical analysis – so how, people naturally ask, can it possibly have any curative effect?

The honest answer is that no one knows, though one theory is that a form of radiation energy is released which stimulates the body's own healing mechanisms. Homoeopaths point out that we do not understand how many modern drugs work, but we do know that a few have unpleasant side-effects. Even though some of the substances from which homoeopathic remedies are made, such as arsenic and mercury, would be poisonous in larger amounts, in homoeopathic doses they are harmless. But with homoeopathic treatment the symptoms will sometimes become worse before they improve.

Homoeopathic medicines can safely be taken in pregnancy – for early morning sickness, for example – and a child could swallow a bottle of most homoeopathic pills with no ill effect. It is possible, however, to have an unpleasant reaction to some remedies if they continue to be taken once the symptoms have gone.

Many homoeopaths are qualified doctors who have done a further year's training in homoeopathy. They may become GPs or work in homoeopathic hospitals (there are only about three of these in the UK), in which case their treatment is available on the NHS, or they may consult privately.

The advantage of consulting a medically qualified homoeopath is that he or she is trained in diagnosis and able to prescribe conventional medicines such as antibiotics when necessary. Most homoeopaths agree that life-threatening conditions are better treated with conventional medicines.

If you consult a homoeopath who is not also a doctor, make sure he or she has done a full homoeopathic training at an approved college: there are some charlatans about. For books, advice, information and a list of practitioners, contact the British Homoeopathic Association, whose address is on p.223.

You can try self-treatment with homoeopathic remedies for everyday complaints. Nelsons and Weleda make a range of homoeopathic remedies, and some, including first-aid or travel kits for everyday ailments – with instructions – are available from specialist chemists such as Ainsworth Homoeopathic Pharmacy (address p.223). I've included a selection of homoeopathic remedies throughout this guide for those interested in trying alternative forms of medicine. I've used the abbreviations – Phos. for phosphorus, for example – which are conventional in homoeopathy. Don't worry if these are unfamiliar – your pharmacist or homoeopath will know what you mean.

There are, however, general instructions that should be followed when treating everyday ailments with homoeopathic remedies. These are the recommendations of the Homoeopathic Development Foundation.

Use the 6th potency, that is, remedies labelled 6c. The suggested dose is two tablets for adults or one tablet for a small child. In acute conditions, give a dose every hour for six doses, then three times a day between meals for three days. In chronic cases, give a dose three times a day between meals until relief is obtained.

Watch the response to each dose. When improvement is evident, increase the interval between doses, continue for two more days, then *stop*. Repeat only if the original symptoms recur. Stop dosing when the condition is cleared.

If the symptoms are aggravated after taking a remedy, stop the medication; when the aggravation has passed, do not repeat the medication. Repeat the medication only if the *original* symptoms recur.

Keep the medicines in a cool, dark place and away from things that smell. Tablets should not be handled. Tip the tablets into the cap of the container and drop them into the mouth. Best results are obtained by chewing or sucking the tablets.

Medicines are best taken apart from food or drink. They should be dissolved on a clean tongue when the mouth is free from the effects of tobacco or strongly flavoured toothpaste.

For more serious conditions the foundation recommends that a qualified homoeopathic physician be consulted

**Herbal Medicine**   Herbs seem to get into everything these days! Of course, they have always added flavour to cooking, and herbal teas, such as rosehip and peppermint, have long been popular. Now, bath oils, shampoos, face and body lotions containing a variety of herbs sell like hot cakes as we are encouraged to believe that all things natural are good for us.

'Herbs' (which include a variety of plants, flowers and even trees) have been used for thousands of years to cure or prevent disease and even today 85% of the world's population is largely dependent on herbal medicine. For a long time no one really understood how or why herbal treatments worked, but more recently scientists have been able to separate many of the active chemical ingredients from healing plants and set up tests to observe their effects.

Some of these substances are now produced synthetically in laboratories and form the basis of modern drugs. For example, digoxin (a heart stimulant) is the synthetic form of the active ingredient of digitalis, found in foxgloves. And salicylates, derived from willow bark, are now produced synthetically as aspirin. However, medical herbalists believe that by isolating and using only the main, active ingredient of the plant, one is losing the benefits provided by the other ingredients working in harmony. They therefore always use the whole plant.

Because of shortage of funds and other difficulties, there have been very few scientific trials using the whole plant (although some research has now proved that feverfew can be effective against migraine). This lack of conclusive evidence is one reason why doctors are sceptical of herbal medicine.

Herbalists say that medicines using the whole plant work in a similar way to foods providing, for example, essential vitamins and minerals – which help protect the body against illness – and enzymes which aid absorption of food.

Some plants have within them a natural antidote to the side-effects a medicinal ingredient could cause, were it extracted and given in isolation. For instance, ephedrine – a drug often prescribed by doctors to relieve bronchial symptoms – comes from the plant *Ephedra sineca* and can cause an increase in blood pressure. But the plant itself includes an ingredient that keeps blood pressure down.

As another example, dandelion leaves are a natural diuretic (that means they stimulate urine production and help to rid the body of excess fluid); they are also rich in potassium, an essential mineral salt. When man-made diuretics are used, the body may excrete too much potassium so that a supplement is needed to replace it. Herbalists can point to many such instances where the ingredients in the plant counterbalance each other.

The herbal remedies available from chemists, health food shops and supermarkets may be helpful for minor problems, but, if symptoms are persistent or severe, consult a registered medical herbalist for a full assessment and tailormade prescription. Looking for the initials MNIMN or FNIMH after the practitioner's name will help you avoid quacks – a professional herbalist (and many people do not realise these exist) will have done four years' training.

Herbal medicine aims not just to treat a particular symptom, but to improve the overall physical and mental well-being of the patient. Diagnosis and treatment based on this holistic approach will include advice on diet and lifestyle, as these may be partly responsible for the symptoms. In fact, herbalism takes so many factors into account that two people with apparently identical symptoms may be given quite different prescriptions. Professional herbalists are trained to use many of the same diagnostic methods as doctors and to refer people on for X-rays and other specialist investigations or treatment, if necessary.

Medicines are usually given in the form of a 'tincture' – a concentrated solution made from suitable herbs which have been soaked in water and alcohol. Sometimes the herbalist provides the actual plants from which to make an 'infusion' (similar to tea) or a 'decoction', whereby the plants are gently simmered for some time and the juices then strained off. Medicinal herbs can also be given as suppositories, ointments and poultices.

It is part of a medical herbalist's training to learn the most effective quantities of each plant to use, but the constituents of the plant can vary, depending on such factors as where it is grown and the time of year it is picked. This means it is impossible to measure accurate dosages, and is another reason that most orthodox doctors still have their doubts about herbal medicine.

Most herbal remedies are safe and mild for children as well as adults, and even the names of many healing plants sound soothing – lemon balm, comfrey, meadowsweet and speedwell, for instance. However, like anything else, they can be harmful if used incorrectly or taken in excess. One man died recently from drinking too much carrot juice – so always follow the instructions carefully.

Some of the more potentially dangerous herbs (like lobelia, an anti-asthmatic) can only be prescribed by medical herbalists and/or doctors. Some, such as devil's claw – a joint and muscle pain-reliever – should be avoided in pregnancy. If you are in any doubt, ask professional advice.

Conventional medicines usually act quickly and are therefore best for acute illness, but they can also cause side-effects. Herbal remedies often take longer to be effective but for simple, common ailments and recurrent problems such as indigestion, constipation, insomnia, eczema, ulcers and headaches, advice and treatment from a medical herbalist could bring relief. Serious side-effects are most unlikely.

Some conventional and herbal medicines work well together but others can interact badly, so always tell your doctor and herbalist about any medicines you are taking. Throughout this guide, I've listed a selection of herbal medicines and remedies available which may help some common ailments. .

For more information about herbal medicine contact the National Institute of Medical Herbalists (address on p.223).


**Dos and Don'ts of Over-the-Counter Medicines**    Every day, six million people in Britain visit pharmacies and a million people ask for advice about symptoms of heartburn and haemorrhoids, corns and constipation. Not only that, more than £580 million a year is now passed over the counter for cough, cold and sore-throat remedies, general and topical analgesics, indigestion and stomach-upset remedies, laxatives, acne treatments, vitamins, eye-care products, anti-diarrhoeal medicines, hay-fever treatments and so on and so on . . .

In every pharmacy an average minimum of 50 people a day will buy an over-the-counter medicine. That's almost three-quarters of a million people a day in Great Britain, so as you can see that self-medication plays a major role in modern health care.

People visit a pharmacy instead of arranging a doctor's appointment for many reasons, including convenience, informality and cheapness (most OTC medicines cost less than the current prescription charge). But there are important guidelines you must follow if OTC medicines are to be used safely.

- Always ask your pharmacist for help.
- Always read the label or packet. This will tell you how much medicine it is safe to take, and when and how to take it. Taking a lot of medicine at once does not mean it will work better or faster, and it can be harmful. If you do take too much medicine, get help quickly – from your doctor, local hospital or chemist – but don't delay. If need be, call an ambulance.
- Take extra care when you give medicine to children, and always keep medicines out of their reach. Be particularly careful when other children are in your house. Never let children play with medicines or even empty medicine bottles.
- If you are pregnant, or think you may be, never take medicines without consulting your doctor.
- Always consult your doctor or pharmacist before taking an OTC medicine if you are already taking medication or have a medical condition.
- Never take an analgesic within four hours of having taken one, even if it is of a different type or brand.
- Tablets or capsules can stick in your throat, so take them with plenty of water while sitting or standing up.
- Swallow capsules whole, unless you are told to open them up.
- If you buy a suppository, unwrap it and follow the instructions. You use it by pushing it into the anus (back passage). A pessary is for use in a woman's vagina (front passage). Remember, your pharmacist is an expert on medicines, so always ask for advice if you are not sure what to do.
- Some medicines may cause drowsiness. If affected don't drive or operate machinery and avoid alcoholic drink. Alcohol or other medicines may change the way your medicine works.
- Aspirin should not be given to children under 12 except by medical advice. There appears to be some connection

between young children taking aspirin and developing Reye's Syndrome – a rare condition (affecting only about seven children in a million) which causes brain inflammation and liver damage. It is not even certain that aspirin is directly implicated, but the possibility is enough to make doctors decide that it is not normally worth the risk. Paracetamol is a safe alternative as a painkiller.

● Don't keep old medicines in your home. Flush them down the toilet, or ask the pharmacist to destroy them for you.

# A–Z of Common Complaints

## ACNE AND SPOTS

Acne is a disorder of the sebaceous glands in the skin which causes spots. It's probably one of the most distressing of common skin conditions and it affects almost all youngsters at some time, although severe cases are rare.

Spots usually appear first when the sufferer is anywhere between the ages of 11 and 15, and disappear when he or she is in the mid to late 20s. In rare and depressing cases they can continue into the late 30s. Acne affects the skin on the face, neck, back and chest and is generally worse in men than in women.

Spots normally occur because of an increase in the production of sebum, the skin's normal oily secretion. Sebum keeps the skin moist and supple – without it, the skin would become dry and might even crack. The over-production of sebum is due to stimulation from a male hormone, androgen, and leads to the shiny skin commonly seen in teenagers. With the increase in this skin grease, the pores in the skin can become blocked and infected by bacteria which thrive on the sebum. This in turn causes spots.

The most common types of acne spots are blackheads, pustules, papules and cysts. Blackheads are very small black spots which usually appear around the nose and chin. They are caused by dead skin cells and sebum collecting in a hair follicle and becoming discoloured by exposure to air. Pustules are inflamed spots with white centres caused by bacterial activity in sebum which has collected in a hair follicle. Papules are inflamed spots. In severe cases, cysts develop – tender, swollen lumps under the skin caused by scar tissue forming around an inflamed area of skin.

Many people, particularly adolescents, suffer deep emotional anguish because of acne. It can become the most important thing in your life, making you embarrassed to meet strangers and even causing you to shy away from friends.

However, there is good news. Help is very often at hand. All sorts of acne treatments are available from your pharmacist. And for the vast majority of sufferers, these can bring remarkable relief. The bad news is that clearing up acne nearly always needs great perseverance. There is no overnight cure and you may have to persist with treatment for several months at a time.

The OTC preparations are topical, that is, they are applied directly to the skin. They fall into various categories. Antibacterial skin-washing creams, lotions and soap can help by reducing bacterial activity in the skin. Antiseptic creams, ointments and soaps can destroy micro-organisms, and abrasives can remove blockages clogging up the skin.

The most common form of treatment available is a keratolytic skin ointment – that means it 'dissolves' the keratin (the top layer of the skin) and encourages peeling of the layer of dead and hardened skin cells that form the skin's surface. These ointments – there are a number of different brands – may contain the keratolytics benzoyl peroxide, sulphur or salicylic acid. Benzoyl peroxide and sulphur also have an antibacterial effect.

If you know you have sensitive skin, or have suffered an adverse reaction to other acne preparations in the past, it's worth applying creams or lotions to a small area of skin for the first few days. If your skin seems to tolerate it, you can then treat larger areas.

Keratolytic preparations often cause soreness of the skin, so they are available in different strengths. Benzoyl peroxide, for instance, is likely to cause a mild burning sensation on the first application, as well as a moderate reddening and peeling of the skin during the first few days. Throughout the first few weeks of treatment, most patients will experience a sudden increase in peeling. This isn't harmful and will subside within a day or two if treatment is temporarily discontinued. Then start treatment again and continue while the acne is kept at bay and the other side-effects remain at non-worrying levels.

But if discomfort such as burning, redness or excessive peeling occurs, stop the treatment temporarily or consult a doctor. Patients with a known sensitivity to this active ingredient shouldn't use products which contain it. Preparations containing benzoyl peroxide shouldn't be used for longer than three months at a time.

It's also worth noting that these products may bleach dyed clothing and fabrics, so use them with care.

If keratolytic ointments don't work for you, consult your doctor, who may recommend an alternative form of treatment such as an antibiotic, or refer you to a specialist dermatologist, who may prescribe Vitamin A-derivative tablets; if you're female the doctor may suggest the use of a contraceptive pill – either a usual one known to be beneficial to the skin or one which, while still having a contraceptive effect, is primarily prescribed for the treatment of acne.

Remember that if you suffer from acne, you should try to avoid worrying about your spots, as this will make them worse. (Easier said than done, I know.) Also restrain yourself from squeezing blackheads and pimples, as this can cause further damage and scarring of the skin, and can also make the spots spread.

Many acne sufferers try to not eat chocolate and other fatty foods, and although there is no real proof that this has any effect on acne, it's worth a try, as a healthy, well-balanced diet with plenty of fresh fruit and vegetables can generally only be good for you. Sunshine can help dry up your spots – but don't overdo it and burn yourself.

**What's Available?**   Acetoxyl 2.5 and 5, Acnegel and

Acnegel Forte, Benzagel 5 and 10, Benoxyl 5 Cream and Benoxyl Creams with Sulphur, Biactol, Brasivol Fine, Cepton, Clearasil Medicated Cleansing Milk and Lotion, Clearasil Medicated Gel and Cream, Panoxyl 2.5, 5 and 10, Sudocrem, Tri-Ac, Ultra Clearasil Acne Treatment Cream, Valderma Range

**My Favourites**   Biactol, Clearasil

**Homoeopathic Remedies**   Belladonna, Hepar. Sulph., Pulsatilla, Silicea, Sulphur

**Herbal Remedies**   Soothene Ointment

## ARTHRITIS
See RHEUMATIC PAIN p.100

## ATHLETE'S FOOT
Athlete's foot (*tinea pedis*) is a fungal infection of the skin which thrives in warm, wet conditions. The skin between the toes becomes red, soggy, itchy, flaky and sometimes smelly. It's not very common in children but is a frequent problem for adolescents and sporty young men and women who use communal changing rooms. The condition will persist until it's treated and, as other people can be infected, prompt attention is required.

Treatment is fairly straightforward. If you suffer from athlete's foot – or as a precaution against it – you should ensure your feet are kept dry. 'Air' them as often as possible, wash them frequently, particularly during hot weather, change socks or stockings daily and avoid walking barefoot in public changing rooms. If you have to use a changing room or communal shower, try wearing sandals to avoid any risk of infection from the floor.

Antifungal creams, sprays or powders are usually very effective. They mainly contain antifungal drugs such as tolnaftate, undecenoic acid, miconazole, dichlorophen or zinc undecenoate and need to be used morning and night after thoroughly washing your feet (always use your own flannel and towel) and removing any loose skin. Rub creams or spray sprays into and around affected skin. Sprinkle powder liberally on to feet, particularly between the toes – it's helpful, too, to dust socks and the insides of shoes before wearing them. Unless the instructions on your medicine advise you differently, continue treatment for a week after all signs of infection have disappeared.

If the condition doesn't clear up in a week or so, you may need a stronger antifungal agent than those available over the counter. Consult your doctor.

**What's Available?**   Daktarin Cream, Spray Powder and Powder, Mycil, Mycota Cream, Spray or Powder, Phytocil Cream and Powder, Tinaderm Powder, Tineafax Powder and Cream

**My Favourites**   Mycil, Mycota Cream

# BACK PAIN

Although one and a half million people in this country are suffering from some degree of back pain at any one time, the majority do get better with no more complicated treatment than bed rest and/or painkilling drugs. In many cases, the pain isn't even bad enough to merit a visit to the doctor, but if you are suffering your first attack of back pain, or if the pain is severe, see your GP before trying any self-medication – the back is a large, complicated area with tens of thousands of nerve-endings, many of which, for different reasons, can cause pain.

When people suddenly develop back pain, they tend to think that they must have 'slipped a disc', imagining the disc to be something like a tap washer. In fact, these interverte-bral discs, as they are called, are firmly attached to the side of each vertebra – the interlinked bones that make up the spine – and it is impossible for them to 'slip'. They are spongy and act as a kind of ball-bearing and shock-absorber whenever the spine moves. When a disc causes trouble it is because a split has developed in its outer layers, allowing some of the soft inner pulp to prolapse – fall – through. This can then press on nearby ligaments or nerves and cause pain which may be severe. A disc (usually in the lumbar – lower back – region) tends to prolapse following some unusual, prolonged and perhaps unaccustomed physical activity. The disc walls are weakened, the back may feel stiff for a few days, and it might then be something quite minor, like a cough or a sneeze, that ruptures the wall.

However, only a tiny proportion – less than 5% – of back pain is caused by disc problems. At some time in their lives, most people will suffer from back pain which could have been prevented. There are many possible causes, the most common being a strain or sprain of one of the ligaments which help to hold the spine together or one of the muscles responsible for its movement.

Sitting or standing for long periods in unsuitable positions can often be blamed. Repetitive work, such as digging or weeding, carried on for too long, is one cause; lifting things incorrectly – while bending at the waist and twisting at the same time, for example – is another. Hours bent over a desk or at a typewriter, especially if the chair does not provide the right back support and the desk is not the correct height, throws a great strain on the back.

It is best to change position frequently, or get up and walk around from time to time, so that the muscles and ligaments get a little exercise – they were not designed to hold the same position for long. Likewise, make sure you give yourself regular breaks from the digging and the weeding!

Sales reps and others who spend hours driving can often benefit from a specially designed car seat with extra back support. Lifting should always be done by bending at the knees like a fork-lift truck, not from the waist like a crane! And combined lifting and twisting movements should be avoided, as these are very likely to strain the back.

Various forms of arthritis also commonly cause back pain. X-rays of people's backs show that osteoarthritis – general wear and tear of the joints – affects nearly everyone over 50 and this may result in pain. Rheumatoid arthritis can sometimes be a cause of inflammation and pain in the back and young men in particular may develop another form of arthritis involving the back – ankylosing spondylitis.

Women are prone to osteoporosis – a thinning of the bones – after the menopause. This may cause one or more of the vertebrae – especially those in the neck – to crumble slightly, resulting in nerve pressure and pain.

One of the reasons for consulting your doctor when you first experience back pain is to exclude less common causes – it often helps just to be assured that there is nothing seriously wrong. But it may still be difficult to pinpoint the exact problem. Relieving the symptoms will then be a question of trial and error, but fortunately most back pain will get better of its own accord within a month – often less.

Bed rest for a few days – longer with disc problems – will help any inflammation to subside. A firm mattress, perhaps placed on the floor or with a large, person-sized board under it, is best. Corsets and collars can provide helpful temporary support, but do not wear a corset for longer than three to four weeks, unless otherwise advised by your doctor, or joints can stiffen up. Heat or ice packs will often relieve pain, but be sure to protect the skin.

Aspirin or other anti-inflammatory and pain-relieving medicines like ibuprofen are most effective, and will also help to relax the tenseness in the muscles which adds to the pain. They need to be taken regularly, as recommended, so that a constant level of pain relief is maintained in the blood and the pain is not allowed to surface. Paracetamol can also ease back pain, although it does not reduce inflammation (see PAINKILLERS p.89 for a list of OTC products containing these ingredients).

None of these medicines should be taken for more than a few days except under a doctor's advice.

Massage (with or without a liniment, or muscle rub) or a

vibrator applied to the painful area can also relax the muscles and be very soothing. A form of physical therapy called the Alexander Technique aims to relax muscles and improve posture by undoing bad sitting and standing habits developed over the years – it will often relieve back ache in the process. Some people find that manipulation of the back by a registered osteopath, chiropractor or physiotherapist will bring relief, but this treatment is best begun within a few days of the onset of the pain. Acupuncture can also be effective when practised by skilled hands.

Exercise, especially swimming, walking and cycling, plays an important part in keeping the muscles and ligaments in good tone. Special exercises designed for the individual by a physiotherapist, especially once the acute pain has subsided, will usually speed recovery and help prevent a relapse.

If the pain is severe – as with lumbago, which afflicts the lower back and is often so agonising that the sufferer is stuck in a stooping position, or especially with sciatica, when the pain is radiating down the leg – stay in bed and call your doctor. If a prolapsed disc is diagnosed or suspected, specialist treatment may be needed.

**What's Available?**    Algipan Rub and Spray, Deep Heat Range, Doan's Tablets, Ibuleve, Massage Balm, Menthol and Wintergreen Heat Rub, PR Freeze Spray

**My Favourites**    Deep Heat Range, Algipan and PR Freeze Spray

**Homoeopathic Remedies**    Aconite, Arnica, Bryonia, Calc. Fluor., Nux. Vom., Rheumasol, Rhus. Tox.,

## BAD BREATH
The really embarrassing thing about bad breath is that all too often you don't become aware of until it's pointed out to you by somebody else. But don't worry – it can affect the best of us, not just heavy smokers or garlic eaters.

Bad breath is medically known as halitosis. It will often be temporary, caused by eating highly spiced foods, for example. Alcohol and cigarettes also give the breath characteristic, unpleasant smells.

But the most likely cause of recurrent bad breath is poor dental hygiene. Plaque – a sticky film of bacteria and other ingredients – can cause decay if allowed to build up around the teeth. It can also cause a gum disease called gingivitis (see GUM DISEASE p.63). The gums will then look inflamed and bleed easily when you brush your teeth. Bad breath is a common accompanying symptom.

Regular brushing of teeth and use of dental floss – a special strong thread or tape which is passed through the spaces between the teeth – combined with a mouthwash (particularly one of the antibacterial mouthwashes containing chlorhexidine) and regular trips to the dentist, will usually bring about a cure.

If your dentist can find nothing wrong and bad breath is persistent, consult your doctor. He can examine you to exclude another common cause – nasal polyps. These are benign growths, readily removed, which can prevent proper drainage in the nose and lead to mild infection. Sinusitis, chronic catarrh, chest infection, digestive problems and constipation are all other possible causes of bad breath.

In fact, any sudden change in diet can be responsible – would-be slimmers have found that a high-protein diet, lacking in carbohydrate and fibre, will often make their breath smell unpleasant. This is likely to be due to lack of fibre in the bowel, causing a change in the 'friendly' bacterial content and its 'cleansing' effect, though no one really knows why this should affect the breath, or if indeed it is the cause of the problem. But charcoal tablets or biscuits could help – probably by absorbing the unpleasant odours, so preventing them from being exhaled.

**What's Available?** Listermint, Listerine Antiseptic, Bragg's Medicinal Charcoal Tablets, Oraldene

**My Favourite**    Listermint

**Homoeopathic Remedies**    Kali. Phos., Merc. Sol.

## BED SORES

If someone who is confined to bed is so ill or paralysed that they don't, or can't, 'turn over' as usual, they risk developing painful bed sores. The skin can crack and weep and, as a result of the continuous pressure on a certain part of the body, the tissues below the skin can 'wear away'. The problem arises because the pressure prevents an adequate amount of blood from getting through to supply the tissues with oxygen and nutrients. This doesn't happen in healthy people because the normal sensations of discomfort – which at their worst become pins and needles – make us turn over or move about, even in our sleep.

These painful areas of skin are also known as pressure sores and usually appear on the buttocks, heels and elbows due to pressure and friction from the bed itself where it is supporting the weight of the body.

Elderly people who have to stay in bed because of illness are particularly vulnerable to bed sores. Often their skin is not as supple or resilient as it used to be and their ageing nerves are not as sensitive to the warning signals that their skin and tissues are becoming numb and they need to move. And the less a patient moves around, the more likely bed sores are to develop. So, if you're looking after an elderly person who is confined to bed, make sure he or she changes position as often as possible.

Barrier creams, zinc and castor oil cream or petroleum jelly, used frequently and well rubbed in, can help protect the skin from irritation. So can talcum powder. It's the regular rubbing that is important. In hospital, when there is any likelihood of such sores developing, the nursing staff will treat those areas already mentioned every four to six hours and turn the patient every two hours.

Should the skin look particularly sore or, even worse, if it is starting to weep, seek help from your doctor or a registered nurse immediately. Once a bed sore has started, it will need regular nursing attention several times a day to clear it up.

**What's Available?**   Sudocrem

**Herbal Remedies**   Hypercal Cream (for cuts and sores)

# BITES AND STINGS

Compared with people in many other countries, we in Britain are lucky in having relatively few biting or stinging insects. Venomous snakes, spiders and such like are also thin on the ground or non-existent.

However, I did say 'relatively' few. That still leaves us with around 33 different kinds of mosquito – commonly known as gnats; about 43 types of midge, six species of wasp, several kinds of bee, not to mention biting horseflies and stinging ants. Jellyfish and poisonous fish can be a hazard too and, especially as more and more of us are taking our holidays abroad, it is important to know what to do if the need arises.

Creatures that sting do so to protect themselves, insects that bite do so to feed. With mosquitoes, midges and horseflies it is only the female that bites; she needs the blood that a good bite gives her in order to rear her young – no consolation to us as we scratch away!

But whether the attack takes the form of a bite or a sting, the result is the same – a hot, red, swollen, itchy area and sometimes, more serious consequences. In the case of a sting, the symptoms are the result of the body's reaction to the poison injected; with a bite, they are due to an anti-clotting substance in the insect's saliva which it injects to make the blood – your blood! – flow more easily as it feeds. Although it is not poisonous, this substance can provoke an allergic-type response around the bite and occasionally throughout the body. Fortunately, mosquitoes in Britain do not carry disease.

When you are bitten early in the season, you are more likely to react and find yourself scratching than later on in the summer. This is because your body gradually develops some tolerance, particularly to your local gnats and midges. However this will not help you when you visit a different area and get bitten by an unfamiliar species!

Some people seem to be more attractive to biting insects than others and individuals differ in how much they react. In general, though, insect-repellants should protect you for about two hours and, if you are bitten, iced water or witch-hazel, calamine lotion or soothing antiseptic creams will usually calm the irritation. Try your best not to scratch either bites or stings, or you may introduce infection.

A bee only stings as a last resort, as it leaves its sting behind and dies soon afterwards. Remove the sting with a fingernail by scraping it out sideways and in the direction the sting is pointing outwards, rather than pinching and pulling it out, as this can squeeze the remaining venom into the skin. To counteract the acid in a bee sting, apply ice-cold water containing a little bicarbonate of soda. Wasp stings are alkaline, so bathe them with a little vinegar in ice-cold water. It doesn't leave its sting behind, just a chemical irritant.

Remedies from the chemist are soothing. They tend to be antihistamine medicines or creams, made specifically for bites and stings, to combat any allergic reactions. They can also reduce more severe swelling and irritation and some contain local anaesthetics to ease pain or irritation. The effects of a sting will usually disappear after a few hours.

However, a few people develop an allergy to wasp or bee stings and can then have an extreme, even life-threatening reaction which may come on only seconds after the sting. The sufferer may feel dizzy and sick, have a runny, itchy nose and eyes and develop a rash. Their limbs may swell, they may have difficulty breathing and even lose consciousness. If any of these symptoms occur after being stung, it is essential to get to a hospital with an accident and emergency unit (casualty department) or to a doctor immediately.

Similarly, for stings in the mouth, multiple stings or if a child under the age of two is stung, it is best to seek medical advice without delay.

Swimming can be a risky business in some waters. If you are stung by a jellyfish you may not feel it at the time but if you develop a painful, swollen area on your body and perhaps a temperature after swimming in the sea, do consult a doctor.

Stinging fish exist even around the British coast and if you tread on one you will certainly know it – the pain is excruciating. The best treatment is to immerse the stung part in very hot – but not scalding – water. This will quickly deactivate the venom.

Snake bites in Britain are unlikely to be too serious – the adder is our only venomous snake. But common first-aid measures such as sucking the wound or making an incision with a razor blade to squeeze out the venom can do more harm than good. It's best just to immobilise the bitten limb with a splint or sling and take the person straight to hospital.

Of course, bites and stings are best avoided altogether and the following tips should help:

● Don't use perfume, hair sprays or aftershave when bees or wasps are around, as they can be attracted by the scent. Bright colours may also attract insects, so wear pale clothes that cover your arms and legs against gnats and midges, especially if you seem prone to insect bites.

● Examine food and sweet drinks before putting them in your mouth and wipe food off your lips if eating out of doors.

● Don't panic if bees or wasps buzz around you and don't hit out at them. Either ignore them or walk away.

● And a final safeguard, wear shoes in the garden and when paddling – particularly in rock pools.

**What's Available?** AllerEze, Anethane Itch-Soothing Cream, Anthisan, Caladryl, Cupal Insect-Bite Cream, Dermacort, Hc45 Hydrocortisone Cream, Lacto Calamine, Lanacane, Lanacort, Lana-Sting Spray and Creme, RBC, Listerine Antiseptic, Dusk Insect-Repellant Cream, Mentholatum Vapour Rub, Solarcaine, Triludan, Triludan Forte, Wasp-Eze, Witch Doctor

**My Favourites**   Anthisan, AllerEze, Triludan

**Homoeopathic Remedies**   Apis. Mel., Pyrethrum Liquid – applied to the area immediately

**Herbal Remedies**   Combudoron Lotion, Dr Valnet's Tegarome, Dr Valnet's Volarome Insect Repellant, Soothene Ointment

## BRUISES

Everyone is familiar with the discolouring of the skin and its deeper tissue as the result of a knock or injury – it often turns blue, purple or black, then fades to yellow after a few days. A bruise is, in fact, caused by blood leaking from damaged blood vessels and then spreading into surrounding tissue. The leaked blood is converted into different chemicals as it is broken down by the body's clearing-away process, which explains the range of colours.

Some people, and especially some women, do bruise more easily than others, even if they are fit and healthy otherwise. This may be because their small blood vessels are easily damaged; alternatively, their blood's ability to clot may be at fault.

If you suffer from a painful bruise, don't rub or massage the bruised area – pressure may make things worse. Bruises are particularly painful if the bruised area lies over a bone. When that's the case the clogged tissues are more tightly stretched. An ice pack, in the form of a cold compress or a packet of frozen peas (peas are very useful because the packet moulds easily to the shape of your body), applied immediately after the knock may help to reduce the bruising; it may also help to numb the pain afterwards.

If it is your leg that is bruised, sitting with your leg resting on something that raises it above your waist and applying a hot water bottle at a comfortably warm temperature may allow the blood to be absorbed back into the bloodstream more quickly.

**What's Available**   Massage Balm, Mentholatum Vapour Rub, Lasonil, PR Heat Spray, PR Freeze Spray, Witch Doctor

**My Favourites**   Lasonil, Witch Doctor

**Herbal Remedies**   Nelson's Arnica Cream

## BURNS (MINOR) AND SCALDS

To treat minor burns, just cool the area in ordinary cold tap water – perhaps by keeping it running on the burned tissues for five or ten minutes – and cover it with a clean, dry dressing. You can also soothe the sore area with creams and sprays specially made for burns and scalds. Most contain an antiseptic and some sprays contain mepyramine maleate, an antihistamine, and benzocaine, a local anaesthetic.

Even a minor burn which is bigger than a 5 cm square should be seen by a doctor. Superficial burns may hurt more than serious, deeper ones. This is because a deeper burn may have destroyed the nerve endings, so you can no longer feel the pain. With much larger burns, the damaged – or absent – skin can no longer prevent the body's water and chemicals from seeping out and evaporating. The subsequent risk of dehydration can be a greater threat than the burn itself.

**What's Available**   Acriflex, Burn Aid Cream, Burneze, Drapolene Cream, Medicaid, Solarcaine, Sudocrem, Witch Doctor

**My Favourites**    Burneze, Acriflex

**Herbal Remedies**    Combudoron Lotion, Dr Valnet's Tegarome

## CALLOUSES

Callouses, areas of hard, thickened skin on the soles and heels of the feet, can be very uncomfortable and make walking quite painful. They are caused by pressure, perhaps from prolonged walking, walking unevenly or something rubbing in a shoe. No one knows why some people are more prone to callouses than others.

They're not contagious and can occur in any area subject to rubbing, such as the ball or heel of the foot. Callouses differ from corns (see p.44) in that they have no core, although in both complaints it is friction which produces the area of thickened skin.

The first step in callous relief is to change your shoes. Make sure they fit well and don't press on the sore parts of your feet. But if your callouses really do cause you discomfort, consult a chiropodist. He or she will probably pare away the hard skin with a scalpel and may recommend a special insole or pad for your shoe or shoes, to relieve any pressure and prevent the callouses recurring.

Some corn paints will soften the hard skin and speed up its removal. It might also help to remove hard skin regularly with a pumice stone and use a good emollient cream to keep your skin soft.

**What's Available**    Compound W, Salatac Gel

## CATARRH
See SINUS PAIN, NASAL CONGESTION AND CATARRH p.102

# CHAPPED OR DRY LIPS

Lips sometimes need more moisture than the rest of the face because they contain no sebaceous glands – glands which secrete sebum, an oily substance that lubricates hair and skin, as well as providing some protection against bacteria. But lips have more melanin, a brown pigment which protects skin against sun.

Melanin can help protect lips from the sun, but not against the drying effects of wind and cold weather. When your lips feel dry, it is natural to lick them to moisturise them. Saliva, in fact, contains a lipase – an enzyme that can 'dissolve' fat. This removes any skin-provided sebum protection as well as any natural moisture. The lips then feel drier than ever and the sufferer, quite reasonably, licks them again – and so the drying process goes on.

If this is happening to you, you must make a conscious effort to stop licking your lips. This may be all you need to do, though regular use of a lip salve to moisturise your lips will help.

If your lips are especially dry, lip creams containing sunscreen agents, emollients or an antiseptic are available. Ask your pharmacist about Vitamin B Complex Tablets (see VITAMINS p.213), as these may be particularly helpful to the elderly.

**What's Available?**   Blistex, Blisteze Cream, Lypsyl, Uvistat Lipscreen Factor 15

**My Favourite**   Blisteze Cream

# CHILBLAINS

Chilblains are reddish-blue discolorations of the skin resulting in burning, itching and pain and usually affecting the toes, fingers and backs of the legs. They can be accompanied by swelling and when severe can ulcerate. They're caused by exposure to cold, which is why you are more likely to develop them in the winter. They affect more women than men and more young women than old.

What appears to happen is that the blood flow through the body, especially to the extremities – fingers, toes and ears – is interrupted as the small blood vessels constrict in the tissues of the sufferer. This is a natural occurrence, as the body automatically supplies less blood to the skin surface in order to retain essential heat deep within the tissues (for the body to function properly, the kidneys, the heart and particularly the brain and the blood have to keep a constant temperature of around the normal 37°C/98.4°F mark).

But with chilblain sufferers this natural defence mechanism causes problems. Those small vessels remain closed up tightly for longer than usual. When fingers or toes are exposed to warmth, the previously under-supplied tissues come 'alive' again as the blood returns to them. Then the body's normal processes react to any damage that's been done. The normal pain that is felt when not enough oxygen gets to the tissue – as with angina of the heart – is not felt when the tissues are very cold, because the nerves are also affected by the cold and do not function properly. When they warm up again and the numbness goes, pain is experienced because the tissues have become more alkaline as they have survived in the absence of an adequate supply of oxygen. That's what causes the pain and itching of chilblains until the local 'chemistry' is restored to normality.

When you get chilblains for the first time, or if they are severe, consult your doctor in order to rule out any more serious problem. Raynaud's Phenomenon, for example, has similar symptoms to chilblains – it is a condition of the hands, fingers and feet which affects people who are unduly sensitive to cold and can result in the tissues themselves becoming permanently harmed.

Treat chilblains by covering them with a loose, dry dressing such as gauze and, if you wish, applying a soothing antiseptic cream. A vapour rub may help increase blood flow, as the rubbing stimulates the circulation. There is also some evidence that one of the B vitamins – nicotinic acid –

helps to prevent chilblains (see VITAMINS p.213).

If you are prone to chilblains, take particular care in cold weather. Dress up snugly in several layers of thin clothing to help insulate your body, and always wear a hat. Probably the best preventive measure of all is to find ways of keeping the extremities warm. Cosy socks and gloves are a must. And why not try battery-heated ones? You can buy them from the Raynaud's Association Trust (address on p.223). You can also improve the circulation in your hands by waving your arms about – movements like those of a cricket bowler are the most effective.

Even if your feet or hands become really cold, never warm them on a radiator, in front of a fire or directly on a hot water bottle - this will only cause you even more pain. Always warm your hands or feet up slowly, perhaps by putting them into lukewarm water.

**What's Available?**    Bengue's Balsam, Chilblain Cream, Zam-Buk Ointment, Mentholatum Vapour Rub, Snow-fire, Sudocrem

**My Favourite**    Snow-fire

**Homoeopathic Remedies**    Apis. Mel., Pulsatilla, Tamus Ointment

**Herbal Remedies**    Soothene Ointment

## COLD, THE COMMON
Each time we have a 'common cold' it could be due to one of a hundred or so different viruses. These spread from person to person by so-called 'droplet infection' – passed on when the sufferer coughs or sneezes, for example. Colds aren't caused by getting wet or cold, but infection is more likely to catch hold if the body's resistance is reduced by chronic illness, fatigue, stress or depression.

Any immunity we develop after catching a particular cold virus is short-lived and may not protect against further infection, as the viruses 'going around' tend to change constantly and none of them can be 'cured' by medicines. They can be fought and destroyed only by your body's natural defences. So those of us who mix with people regularly can expect to meet and succumb to two or three colds a year.

Typical cold symptoms will be familiar to nearly everyone – the streaming eyes, running and/or blocked-up nose, headache and dry, tickly cough. But although, singly or in combination, they can be very unpleasant, they'll normally improve within a few days and for a straightforward cold, it's not usually necessary to consult a doctor.

If you have a cold, drink plenty of fluids, take aspirin or paracetamol to relieve feverish symptoms – paracetamol is best for children (see PAINKILLERS p.89 for products containing these ingredients). Tepid sponging may cool and soothe children. As long as they have plenty of liquids, don't worry too much if they refuse to eat – their appetites recover very quickly. But do call your doctor if your child develops a high fever, persistent coughing, wheezing, earache or sickness.

For adults, of course, there's a bewildering array of over-the-counter preparations for the common cold. While you cannot treat the virus itself and the 'cold cures' won't speed up recovery, you can get some relief from the effects by taking a mild painkiller as mentioned above, or you can try one of the many cold treatments available these days – which normally contain aspirin or paracetamol anyway. Always follow instructions strictly and never take more than one product at a time.

This is most important since a medicine like paracetamol can build up in the body if you continue to take it over many days or even weeks – you are effectively taking an overdose. And though it's very rare, such a build-up can occasionally cause a tragedy.

Both aspirin and paracetamol will bring down a temperature as well as relieving pain. Other ingredients of cold treatments are likely to be a decongestant to relieve nasal congestion or catarrh, an antihistamine to control the allergic-like symptoms of a cold – streaming eyes, for instance – and sometimes the stimulant caffeine. Many also contain Vitamin C, which some people feel is beneficial.

Many cold-sufferers take large doses of Vitamin C, but I've never seen any evidence that it does any good. In fact, I think that if you take extra Vitamin C, your cold may go in seven days. Without it, it could take as long as a week! Fortunately, it is one of the vitamins which can be taken in large doses without apparent harm, but why take the risk? It really depends on what you feel about it. You pays your money or you takes your chance, and I prefer to take my chance.

Bear in mind that some over-the-counter cold cures may be unwise for pregnant women, for people with diabetes, high blood pressure, heart or thyroid disease and stomach ulcers. As with all medicines, if you do have any medical condition, or are taking other medicines, you should check with your doctor or pharmacist before taking self-medication.

Some products may cause drowsiness, too. If you are affected, do not drive or operate machinery and avoid alcoholic drink. Children taking medicines which may make them drowsy should never be left on their own, except in a safe place – like bed.

There are occasions, however, when you may need to consult a doctor about your cold. If symptoms persist, or if you already have a chest condition – chronic bronchitis, for example – it is best to see your doctor at the first sign of a cold or flu. You may need antibiotics to prevent the development of secondary bacterial infections which could cause further lung damage.

As well as those with existing chest problems or heart disorders, the very young and the very old are especially at risk from complications as a result of a cold or similar infection. They should be watched carefully in case their symptoms worsen. The ageing immune (disease-fighting) system is less effective at combating infection and the elderly are therefore particularly vulnerable.

So how will you know when to call a doctor? Coughing up green, as opposed to clear, sputum is a sure sign that a secondary bacterial infection has developed and antibiotics may then be helpful. Likewise if the cough is very bad. Other symptoms to watch for include streaks of blood in the sputum, breathlessness, wheezing (which may indicate asthma), croup, 'tightness' or pain in the chest and blueness around the lips.

It is also wise to consult a doctor if the patient's temperature, pulse and breathing rate rise and he or she seems generally unwell. Elderly people can develop pneumonia quite untypically, by suddenly becoming confused but having only minor chest symptoms, so be on the look out for this and call the doctor without delay if you are concerned. In fact, real concern is a good criterion for asking a doctor's opinion in any circumstances – if only for reassurance – and this applies as much to symptoms associated with the 'common cold' as to anything else.

**What's Available?**    Actifed Syrup or Tablets, Benylin Day and Night Cold Treatment, Benylin Mentholated Linctus, Bronalin Dry Cough Elixir, Bronalin Paediatric Linctus, Bronchial Catarrh Pastilles, Catarrh-Ex, Coldrex Tablets and Hot Drinks, Contac 400, Cupal Baby Chest Rub, Dimotapp Elixir, Dimotapp Elixir Paediatric, Dimotapp L.A., Fennings Lemon-Flavoured Mixture, Flurex Bedtime Medicine, Flurex Hot Lemon Syrup, Flurex Tablets or Capsules, Junior Lemsip, Lemsip, Lemsip Cold Relief Capsules, Odourless Garlic One-A-Day, Sanatogen One-A-Day Garlic Perles, Snuffle Babe, Vapex Inhalant, Vicks Coldcare, Vicks Vapo-Lem, Vicks Vapo Rub

**My Favourites**    Benylin Day and Night Cold Treatment, Actifed, Contac 400, Vicks Vapo Rub

**Homoeopathic Remedies**    Aconite, Gelsemium, Merc. Sol., Nat. Mur.

**Herbal Remedies**   During the last few years an enormous amount of research into garlic's health-promoting properties and its chemistry has resulted in renewed interest in the way it can help the body's natural systems. Taken as a regular part of the daily diet garlic may help to maintain a healthy heart and circulation. It is also used as a herbal remedy for the relief of catarrh and symptoms of rhinitis and of the common cold.

Herbelix Specific, Hofels Garlic Perles and One-A-Day Garlic Perles, Hofels Garlic Parsley Tablets, Lustys Garlic Perles, Olbas Pastilles, Shen Chinese Garlic Tablets, Cirkulin Garlic Pearls

# COLD SORES

Although cold sores are not usually a serious condition in themselves, they can cause considerable embarrassment and distress – and, inevitably, they tend to arrive at the most inopportune times. The typical little blisters which develop into weeping sores usually appear in groups around the lips but may also occur on other parts of the face. If precautions are not taken, the virus responsible can also be spread to others, or to other parts of the body – the eye for example – with potentially more serious results.

Cold sores are caused by the Herpes Simplex Type 1 virus, one of the herpes group of viruses, others of which cause chicken pox, shingles and glandular fever. A slightly different strain of the same virus, known as Type II, is the one usually responsible for outbreaks of herpes blisters around the genital area, although Type I may be the culprit here, too.

These viruses have one important thing in common – after the first infection, they can lie dormant, causing no symptoms, in the nerve cells of the affected area. Under certain conditions, however, they may be reactivated and track up the same nerves to the same area of skin to produce further outbreaks of blisters. It is estimated that about half the adults in this country are carriers of Type 1 herpes. Most of them will have had their first, often symptomless and undetected infection in early childhood. Many will never have another attack, some may have one after an interval of several years and a small percentage will have recurrent episodes every few months.

Various factors can contribute to reactivating the virus – exposure to sunlight, some infections and being generally 'run down' are amongst them. For a woman, an outbreak of cold sores is more likely during menstruation. However, with each new outbreak, the body produces further anti-bodies which accumulate to fight the virus – this means that, in time, outbreaks tend to lessen in both frequency and severity.

Cold sores are highly contagious while the blisters are present. The virus is also found in the saliva of the sufferer and can be spread to others – so keep your kisses until the blisters have gone.

You can infect vulnerable parts of your own body, via the fingers, if you touch the sores and do not wash your hands afterwards. Any area of broken skin is especially susceptible. It is particularly important to avoid touching the blisters and then rubbing the eyes, as the virus may be transferred and cause an ulcer on the delicate membrane covering the eye – if this is not diagnosed and treated soon enough, it can damage the sight.

Mothers with cold sores should take extra care and wash their hands frequently, and always after applying medica-tion – babies and toddlers are extremely vulnerable to cold sores as they won't have had time to build up their antibodies. It is also important to keep the flannels, towels, eating and drinking utensils of the sufferer separate from those of the rest of the family.

With both types of herpes, close physical contact is needed before others are infected, so if reasonable precautions are taken during the week or so that the blisters last, there should be little cause for concern. The virus cannot be passed on while it is dormant and producing no symptoms, but whenever you're infectious it is essential to protect others.

Many sufferers from recurrent cold sores notice definite warning symptoms before an outbreak – a 'prickly' feeling in the area of skin usually affected, for instance. If you apply an antiviral ointment or solution prescribed by your doctor during this phase, you can shorten the duration of the outbreak considerably. Cold-sore creams from the pharmacist can also help. These sometimes contain ammonia, small doses of disinfectant, an antiseptic or local anaesthetic.

A simple old wives' remedy is to apply cold coffee to the area on a piece of clean cotton wool every two or three hours and allow it to dry. It may sound primitive, but it appears to work for many people, so it is worth trying if a doctor or pharmacist isn't available. Other than this, the sores should just be kept clean and dry.

A regular, well-balanced diet will help maintain your general health and may therefore prevent attacks. So too may a good sun-blocking cream applied liberally to the lips before and during a concentrated period of sunbathing. But there is no cure for cold sores and if you are prone to them, keep a supply of cream in your medicine cupboard so that you can start the treatment when the warning symptoms first occur. Eventually you will develop your own natural resistance and cold sores should then become a thing of the past.

**What's Available?**    Blisteze, Cupal Cold Sore Ointment, Cupal Cold Sore Lotion

**My Favourite**    Blisteze

# COLIC
Colic in babies is caused by bubbles of gas or air which become trapped in the immature digestive system. The consequent pain makes the baby cry, often inconsolably, and draw his or her legs up in pain. Problems with colic often

appear when the baby is about three weeks old. They can be very wearing for the parents as well as the child, but don't despair, they usually stop of their own accord at about three months.

There are ways you can help soothe your colicky baby. Rocking or cuddling should help, and a car journey or pram ride will often send the baby off to sleep. Giving the age-old but new-formulated remedy, gripe water, has soothed many a baby's mother and sometimes the baby too!

There are new gripe mixtures available which are alcohol- and preservative-free. Gripe water can relieve the colicky pains, wind and troublesome hiccups. But always ask your health visitor or doctor for advice the first time your baby screams inconsolably.

**What's Available?**   Dentinox Infant Colic Drops, Fennings Gripe Mixture, Nurse Harvey's Gripe Mixture

**My Favourite**   Dentinox

**Homoeopathic Remedies**   Chamomilla 3 × Drops or Pillules

## CONJUNCTIVITIS
See STICKY EYES p.109

## CONSTIPATION
With several million pounds being spent each year on laxatives, constipation is clearly a very common problem, though women are three times more likely to suffer from it than men. Yet in healthy people it is an ailment that is almost entirely preventable by simple, natural methods and laxatives should rarely be needed.

Many people consider themselves constipated if they do not 'go' regularly every day. But we all have our own natural rhythm. Some people go twice a day, some people every two or three days and both are quite normal if the habit is regular. In fact, bowel habits naturally vary and, as long as the motion is soft and well-formed and the bowel movement effortless, it doesn't matter if it occurs twice a day or twice a week.

Medically speaking, being constipated usually means passing hard, pellet-like stools with considerable effort and straining. Symptoms also include a bloated abdomen and a feeling of fullness. Being 'irregular' is not the same as constipation and is not necessarily a problem. It's only if your normal bowel habit changes for no good reason for more than a week or two, or if you notice any blood or mucus in your stools, that you should go to your doctor for advice.

Because of the straining associated with it, chronic constipation can lead to other unpleasant conditions such as piles, hiatus hernia and diverticuli – small 'blow outs' in the lining of the bowel which, if they become inflamed, develop into painful diverticulitis. So it makes sense to avoid becoming constipated if possible. The easiest way to do this is to increase the amount of fibre – roughage – in your diet.

Fibre, the undigestible part of cereals, fruit and vegetables, is nature's laxative and most of us would benefit from eating at least half as much again as we do at present. The bulk it provides gives the bowel muscles something to work on and helps to speed up the elimination of food waste after the nutrients have been absorbed during digestion. Fibre swells with the water it absorbs from the gut, so this also helps to produce a soft, well-formed motion.

Many people believe that just eating a bit of extra fruit will soon cure constipation, but this is unlikely to be enough. In fact, bran, the outer husk of cereals, is the richest source of undigestible fibre – far more so than any fruit or vegetables. Wheat bran is the richest source of all.

The refining process used to produce white bread and flour, for example, removes this husk, so an easy way to increase your fibre intake is to eat more wholemeal bread flour and pastas. A daily helping of bran breakfast cereal is another excellent way and natural, uncooked bran can also be sprinkled into soups and stews. Porridge oats, brown rice, baked beans, peas, lentils and sweet corn are high in fibre too. Fruit – unpeeled is best – vegetables and nuts contain a different kind of fibre, and for maximum benefit, eat a good variety of all types of fibre-containing foods regularly.

Expectant mothers and the elderly should avoid eating large quantities of uncooked bran as it may interfere with absorption of minerals such as iron and calcium. Other types of edible fibre can be taken as required.

Contrary to popular belief, too much fibre in your diet will not give you diarrhoea. A *sudden* increase in fibrous food, however, may cause flatulence until the body adjusts, so it is best to make changes gradually.

Remember also that putting off going to the loo can lead to a loss of your usual bowel reflexes, which in turn will cause constipation. Always make a conscious attempt to go to the loo promptly whenever you feel the need.

Many people do rely on laxatives, and although this is not particularly harmful, it is a little unwise, especially if you take them all the time. They can interfere with the normal digestive processes and essential nutrients in the diet pass straight through instead of being absorbed into the body, where they would be of benefit. The risk of vitamin and mineral deficiencies is therefore one good reason not to adopt this practice.

If you do feel the need for laxatives in cases of short-term constipation, your pharmacist can advise you and suggest a suitable one. Laxatives go to work on the large intestine either by speeding up the progress of faecal matter passing through the bowel or by increasing its bulk. Stimulant laxatives such as senna make the bowel muscle contract to hurry the faeces along and bulk-forming laxatives such as ispaghula soak up water in the bowel to increase volume and make stools softer.

The laxative phenolphthalein is often referred to as a stimulant laxative. What happens is this. As food passes down the alimentary canal, the stomach and small intestine require water in order to digest it. At this stage, the contents of the alimentary tract are fluid. There is a water conservation mechanism in the colon, where excess water is re-absorbed into the body, and this can cause constipation. The stimulant effect of phenolphthalein is that it stimulates the onward squeezing movements of the colon, which hampers water absorption because the bulk within the colon is moved on too quickly.

Other laxatives contain liquid paraffin, a lubricant which makes the faeces softer and easier to pass. These should not be taken less than two hours after a meal, since there is a theoretical risk that the liquid paraffin content could interfere with the absorption of some essential vitamins.

If your bowels are very sluggish, your doctor or pharmacist may recommend extra fibre in the form of tablets, or pleasant fruit-flavoured drinks, such as Fybogel or Regulan, made from the husk of the ispaghula plant. Plenty of watery drinks and some daily exercise will also help to keep the bowels moving.

So if you often find yourself resorting to laxatives, first check with your doctor that there is no underlying medical cause for your constipation – an underfunctioning thyroid gland is one possibility – and ask if a higher fibre diet would help you. If, with your doctor's agreement, you then start to eat considerably more of the foods I have mentioned, you should soon find you are saving money on laxatives and can spend it more enjoyably and healthily on food! You may even lose some weight, too – fibrous foods are filling but usually low in calories and therefore slimming!

**What's Available?**   Agarol, Alophen, Andrews Liver Salt, Bonomint, Brooklax, Califig, Correctol, Dulcolax, Ex-Lax Pills and Tablets, Laxoberol, Metamucil, Milk of Magnesia, Mil-Par, Nylax, Petrolagar, Regulan, Reguletts, Senlax, Sure-Lax

**My Favourites**   Senlax, Ex-Lax, Dulcolax

**Homoeopathic Remedies**    Nux. Vom., Silicea, Sulphur

**Herbal Remedies**    Dual-Lax, Lustys Herbalene, Pileabs Tablets

# CORNS

Corns are small lumps of hard skin on the toes, especially over the bony prominences, or on the sides of the feet. They are caused by friction or continual pressure from poorly fitting shoes. The constant rubbing causes a layer of thickened skin to develop which is gradually pushed inwards to form a nucleus or core. It eventually becomes painful when this core presses on a nerve.

There are several types of corn, of which the most common are the hard corn, soft corn and seed corn. A hard corn is a raised shiny dome of whitish or pale yellow thickened skin with a hard cone-shaped centre. It has no root and usually develops on top of the toe joints.

A soft corn appears in the damp area between the toes where the skin surfaces rub together. It is paler and softer than a hard corn. A seed corn is similar in structure but is found on the heel or ball of the foot where the skin can be dry and not very elastic. It is the least painful of the three and often feels like grit in the skin.

To ease discomfort you can soften the hard skin with one of the corn treatments available. Preparations for treating corns usually contain keratolytics such as salicylic acid, to encourage the layer of hardened skin cells to peel off. Be careful to keep any of these solvents off the skin surrounding the corn. If solvent accidentally gets on the normal skin, wash it off immediately.

When treating corns between the toes, hold the toes apart until the solvent has completely dried – putting cotton wool between the toes is a good way of doing this. To prevent further pressure on the corns, buy some small spongy rubber rings to put around them. Beware of corn plasters – if applied incorrectly, they can do more harm than good.

If you frequently have painful corns, it is best to visit a chiropodist. Look in the Yellow Pages for chiropodists with the letters SRCh MChS after their names.

People with diabetes should always consult their doctor about foot problems, since they are more likely to pick up infections in these sore areas. Because diabetic sufferers tend to have poor circulation, they should avoid wearing tight socks or shoes which could reduce the blood flow to the feet.

We all need to look after our feet – an incredible 90% of all foot problems are caused by wearing ill-fitting or the 'wrong' shoes, so do take time to choose new shoes carefully.

**What's Available?**   Carnation Corncaps, Cupal Corn Solvent and Pads, Freezone Liquid, Salatac Gel

**My Favourite**   Carnation Corncaps

**Herbal Remedies**   Lanes Balto Foot Balm

# COUGHS
A cough is not an illness in itself, but a symptom. Although it can be irritating and often embarrassing, it is the body's natural response to any foreign body, congestion or irritation in the lungs or throat. The irritation may be due to things like air pollution or cigarette smoke, but in a great many cases it turns out to be the result of a cold or flu virus.

Sometimes, however, coughing signals a more serious disorder in the respiratory tract. So it is extremely important to seek medical advice for any cough that lasts for longer than a few days or if there are streaks of blood in any mucus you cough up. Coughing up green sputum probably signifies a bacterial infection.

Coughs can be treated with cough suppressants or expectorants. Cough suppressants – as the name suggests – are medicines that suppress the symptom, the cough itself, without tackling the underlying cause. They reduce the frequency and intensity of a cough by acting on the part of the brain that controls the coughing reflex, or at the site of irritation in the throat. These may help if you have a dry, hacking cough. Dry coughs occur when there is irritation but little phlegm in the larynx at the top of the windpipe, or in the pharynx, the cavern between the mouth and nose at the top and the oesophagus (gullet) and trachea (windpipe) below. This irritation stimulates the cough reflex which is the body's natural response.

Expectorants relieve chesty coughs, the type you often get as a result of a cold or flu. These medicines claim to loosen the 'debris' or phlegm in order to make it easier to cough up.

There is certainly a bewildering range of cough medicines available in any pharmacy. Some simply contain soothing substances such as honey and glycerine to act on the throat's surface, together with pleasant-tasting flavourings and tiny doses of antiseptics. Some are sugar-free so that they can be taken by those suffering from diabetes, and will not cause tooth decay. Others are specially designed for children and some are even animal fat-free! Still others contain decongestants to help clear nasal passages or antihistamines to help ease allergy-like symptoms like the nasal congestion, sneezing and watery eyes that may accompany a cough.

Some cough medicines can cause drowsiness. If a medicine makes you drowsy do not drive or operate machinery. And avoid alcoholic drink. Children being given cough medicines which may cause drowsiness should not be left on their own.

If you do have an irritating cough and want something to relieve it, describe your cough to your pharmacist and take his or her advice. You don't want to buy something that may make your cough worse. As always, you should tell your pharmacist if you are taking any other medication, have a medical condition or are pregnant or think you may be.

Despite the enormous number of cough remedies available, there is disagreement as to their value. They may give temporary relief to a tickly throat and taste pleasant, even soothing, but they may or may not be any more effective than a honey drink you have made yourself or inhaling steam to ease congestion. Doctors are sometimes reluctant to prescribe cough suppressants because coughing is a protective reflex; repeated bouts of coughing can be distressing, however, so soothing medication may be needed.

When patients are well in themselves but the troublesome cough is keeping them awake at night and to no good purpose, then I'm in favour of cough suppressants. One instance when they can really be useful is when a person is over the worst of whooping cough, but the cough is persisting after the infection has past – as it sometimes can, for weeks afterwards.

**What's Available?** Actifed Compound Linctus, Actifed Expectorant, Benylin, Benylin with Codeine, Benylin Dry Cough Linctus, Benylin Children's Cough Linctus, Bronal Cough Balsam, Bronalin Dry Cough Elixir, Bronalin Paediatric Linctus, Bronalin Expectorant Linctus, Bronchial Catarrh Pastilles, Children's Cough Pastilles, Copholco, Copholcoids, Cupal Baby Cough Syrup, Dimotane Co, Dimotane Co Paediatric, Dimotane Expectorant, Do-Do Expectorant, Do-Do Tablets, Famel Honey and Lemon Cough Pastilles, Famel Expectorant, Famel Original, Famel Linctus, Franolyn Sed, Franolyn Expectorant, Gee's Linctus Pastilles, Lemsip Expectorant, Lemsip Linctus, Meltus Adult Dry Cough Elixir, Meltus Adult Expectorant, Meltus Baby Cough Linctus, Meltus Junior Expectorant, Night Cough Pastilles, Pavacol-D, Pholcodine Cough Pastilles, Robitussin Cough Soother Adult and Junior, Robitussin Expectorant Plus, Robitussin Expectorant, Sudafed Linctus, Throaties, Vicks Cough Syrup – Expectorant, Vicks Vaposyrup for Dry Coughs

**My Favourite** Benylin

**Homoeopathic Remedies** Aconite, Bryonia, Drosera

**Herbal Remedies**    Garlic (see COMMON COLD p.37), Olbas Pastilles


# CRADLE CAP

Cradle cap is a harmless condition resembling dandruff that is extremely common in young babies. It usually appears during the first three months of a baby's life, but can also affect toddlers and young children. If your baby develops cradle cap, you may first of all notice a little scurf on his or her head, followed by the appearance of yellowish or brownish greasy-looking scales of thickened skin which stick to the scalp. These patches sometimes appear over the whole head, sometimes just in small areas. Some specialists believe the crusts are due to excess production of sebum – grease from the sebaceous glands – in response to the mother's hormones.

Although it can be unsightly, cradle cap is unlikely to do your baby any harm. It usually disappears on its own after a few months. To ease it you can rub the baby's head with baby oil or olive oil and leave for 24 hours. Comb the hair gently, then wash the flakes of skin away. Alternatively, treat cradle cap with specially formulated gentle, medicated shampoo until the scalp is clear.

If you are worried and the cradle cap persists despite treatment, do seek the advice of your doctor or health visitor.

**What's Available?**    Capasal Therapeutic Shampoo, Cradocap Shampoo, Dentinox Infant Cradle Cap Shampoo

**My Favourite**    Cradocap


# CRAMP

Cramp is a common problem which can be extremely painful. It is a sudden, violent contraction of a muscle which makes the muscle become hard and tense. It's usually caused

by exercise, especially unaccustomed exercise, or a prolonged period of sitting, lying or standing in an awkward
position. Some people wake at night with cramp in their feet
or legs. Attacks usually occur in bouts which last from a few
days to a number of weeks, and there are often several
weeks between each series of attacks.

No one really knows what causes cramp. It may occasionally be the result of a poor blood supply due to the furring up
of the arteries – this is especially likely with elderly sufferers.
But in the majority of cases, it's worth trying all the cramp
remedies, in the hope that one of them will do the trick. It is
not possible to be more specific about a 'cure' when no one
knows the cause of the problem.

With the most common sort of cramp, in the calf muscles,
try this. Stand facing a wall and at arm's length from it. Place
the flat of your hands against the wall and gently bend
forward from the ankles so that your calves are gently but
comfortably stretched. Do this standing 'press-up' six times
on three separate occasions throughout the day and continue it for ten days. If it works, keep doing it six times once
a day to keep the cramp at bay. If it doesn't work, stop after
ten days. This will stop me from worrying that you are
continuing forever, wearing out the wallpaper to no good
effect!

**What's Available?**   Crampex, Massage Balm

## CUTS AND GRAZES
You can treat most cuts and grazes at home quite safely, but
always wash your hands first, if possible. Clean the cut by
holding it under running water, or by gently wiping it with
an antiseptic wipe or cotton wool soaked in warm water. It's
best to use a fresh piece of cotton wool for each wipe. Some
small cuts will still bleed quite profusely at first, so if this is
happening after a few minutes, you'll need to apply pressure
to stem the flow. Press a pad, a clean tissue for example,
firmly over the cut for a few minutes.

If you like to use plasters and antiseptic ointments on cuts and grazes, fine – it will do no harm. Personally, I prefer not to use ointments and I use plasters mainly to keep dirt out of the wound. When that isn't necessary or the injury is small, it will heal up nicely if left alone.

If a cut is very large or deep, if it has rugged or gaping edges, if something is embedded in it or if it is a deep cut with only a small opening in the skin (this might happen if the culprit is a rusty nail, for example) always seek medical help.

**What's Available?**   Acriflex Burn Aid Cream, Dettol, Drapolene Cream, Lanacane, Medicaid, Savlon, Savlon Dry, Solarcaine, Sudocrem, Witch Doctor

**My Favourite**   Savlon

**Herbal Remedies**   Dr Valnet's Tegarome, Nelsons Calendula Cream (to soothe abrasions), Hypercal Cream, Soothene Ointment

## CYSTITIS

Cystitis is an inflammation of the bladder lining and the urethra – the tube down which urine is excreted from the bladder. It is one of the most common complaints suffered by women, and estimates suggest that more than half the women in the UK contract cystitis at some time (though it occasionally afflicts men and children too). If you have had it, you will certainly wish to avoid a recurrence. Some women experience attacks several times a year and an unfortunate few are seldom free of the problem.

A woman's anatomy makes her particularly prone to cystitis. Unlike a man's, her urethra is very short and the normally harmless germs around the anus are easily able to track upwards to the bladder, whose natural defences may be unable to cope with them. Some people say they suffer more from cystitis when they are 'run down'. It is likely that they feel run down because there is a niggling infection there which doesn't cause local symptoms all the time, but causes the sufferer to feel under par – that is, run down. From time to time, however, the local symptoms will present themselves.

Inflammation then develops and often spreads to the urethra – a condition known as urethritis – which results in the typical burning pain as urine is passed. The urine is often dark brown and strong smelling; it may also contain traces of blood. The sufferer has a constant urge to 'spend a penny' even though there is little or nothing to pass. A slight temperature, nausea, a dragging feeling in the lower abdomen and tenderness over the bladder are also common, as is a general feeling of being unwell. However, cystitis is by no means always due to an infection. The delicate lining of the urethra and/or the bladder can, in those susceptible, react to irritants such as scented soaps, powders, vaginal deodorants, bath oils and the detergents used to wash clothes. Some people are sensitive to highly spiced foods, strong tea, coffee, alcohol and fruit juices. Friction or bruising during lovemaking can also inflame the tissues, as the urethra is just above the vaginal entrance – a lubricant jelly may then help by overcoming any dryness. Hormone replacement therapy or oestrogen cream may be more effective after the menopause.

Germs can also be inadvertently 'helped' into the urethra during intercourse. Inserting tampons can do this too, as can wiping yourself from back to front (instead of front to back) after a bowel movement. The main germ which causes trouble here and after sexual intercourse is one called *Escherichia coliform*, more commonly known as *E. coli*. It lives in the bowel, where it is harmless, but if it makes its way to the vagina or urethra it can cause problems.

Thrush infection, perhaps aggravated by wearing tight-fitting trousers, is another possible cause of symptoms. It is important, too, to pass urine as soon as you feel the need and to empty your bladder completely each time by squeezing out every last drop – a reservoir of urine can make a fertile breeding ground for germs.

So, if you are prone to cystitis, always wash around your vaginal area and 'spend a penny' both before and after making love. Having sex with a full bladder, or bowel for that matter, means bruising is more likely to occur, which can also encourage cystitis. Ask your partner to wash daily, too.

Try to drink at least three or four pints of water every day to flush out any germs and prevent them settling. It has been suggested that a glass or two of cranberry juice a day may also help to keep cystitis at bay. No one knows quite why, but some Americans swear by it.

If symptoms do develop, neutralising the acidity is a worthwhile first line of treatment, since as many as two out of three sufferers won't actually have any infection and the symptoms should therefore settle in a day or so using this method alone. Start immediately symptoms appear by drinking a pint of water with a teaspoonful of bicarbonate of soda added – unless you suffer from high blood pressure, or heart or kidney trouble, in which case consult your doctor first. Drink a pint of this mixture every hour for three hours, interspersed with other soft drinks. This will change the urine from acid to alkaline and relieve the pain, but it is not something I would recommend too often, as an excess of bicarbonate of soda, especially in a sufferer whose kidneys are not working properly, could lead to side-effects such as a rise in blood pressure.

Alternatively you could take potassium citrate or a specially formulated, pleasant-tasting medicine from the chemist. These medicines mainly contain sodium citrate to make the urine less acid and are usually meant to be taken regularly for 48 hours. Such treatments can be very helpful, but if symptoms persist after the 48 hours are up, you should see your doctor – take a specimen of urine with you in a clean, screw-topped jar. If infection is found or suspected, antibiotics are usually effective but be sure to complete the course. You should not need to repeat treatments often, either.

If your symptoms come back regularly, see your doctor

for advice. Just occasionally, if cystitis is a constant problem, there may be a rarer cause for which further investigations will be necessary.

Over-the-counter treatments for cystitis should not be taken by children except on medical advice, nor if you are pregnant or breast-feeding, if you have heart disease or high blood pressure, if you have had any kidney disease or if you are on a low salt diet.

Other helpful measures include rest in bed and a hot water bottle placed over your abdomen; your preferred painkiller will also make you feel better.

**What's Available?**    Cymalon, Cystoleve, Cystopurin

**My Favourite**    Cymalon

# DANDRUFF AND SEBORRHOEIC DERMATITIS

Dandruff is a condition rather like acne which, although not serious, can be acutely embarrassing to those who suffer from it and a source of amusement to those who don't. It is also the most common cause of itching of the scalp, but is not a sign of general ill health.

Normally, everyone's skin cells, including those on their scalp, are replenished about every 28 days and the top layer regularly shed in minute, usually unnoticeable pieces. In dandruff sufferers, this process may be speeded up and the particles shed are larger and easily seen. With milder forms of dandruff, sometimes known as scurf, the flakes of skin are dry and white and tend to clump together in the hair. Touching the hair – which most people do many times a day without realising it – dislodges the fragments and they fall on to the shoulders, looking like a white powder.

This type of dandruff can usually be controlled by washing the hair two or three times a week with a medicated, anti-dandruff shampoo. These often contain tar, sulphur or salicylic acid to soften and help loosen scale and scalp debris. Other anti-dandruff shampoos for more severe cases contain zinc pyrithione or selenium sulphide to reduce the development of dandruff by slowing down the growth of skin cells, as well as having mild antifungal properties.

There is, however, a more severe form of dandruff called seborrhoeic dermatitis of the scalp, which may not respond to these shampoos. It can occur on other parts of the body, too, and may be very difficult to treat effectively.

Seborrhoeic dermatitis can affect both children and adults. On a baby's scalp it is known as cradle cap (see p.48) and the condition often also appears as a nappy rash for which your doctor can prescribe a cream. For adults and older children, Capasal Therapeutic Shampoo may help, as it 'dissolves' the skin flakes but also contains a moisturiser to protect the skin from dehydration.

When they occurred in adults, both seborrhoeic dermatitis and other forms of dandruff used to be thought to be due to over-production of sebum. Diet, hygiene, climate and stress were also thought to play a part. However, recent research has shown that it is the sufferer's over-reaction to a minute, fungus-like organism called *Pityrosporum ovale*. It is the reaction to the fungus, rather than the fungus itself, that causes the scalp's top layer of skin to flake off as dandruff, or gives rise to the symptoms of seborrhoeic dermatitis.

In this condition, which is most common in young men but can affect women, too, the flakes of skin are large, yellow and oily. The skin on the scalp becomes red, inflamed and soggy, especially around the edges, and may be infected by other germs. Eyelashes, eyebrows, skin folds on either side of the nose and behind the ears can all be affected, as can other parts of the body, such as the chest, armpits, breasts and groin.

Neither dandruff nor seborrhoeic dermatitis is catching, because, as I said, it is not the fungus itself that produces the symptoms – as it is with athlete's foot, for instance – but an over-reaction to it which only occurs in susceptible people. The fungus itself is around all the time. Why some people and not others have this susceptibility isn't known.

If you find your dandruff cannot be controlled by medicated shampoos from your pharmacist, do consult your doctor, as there are now effective treatments which he or she can prescribe. The same advice applies if you think you have seborrhoeic dermatitis. Your doctor's examination will exclude other possible skin conditions such as psoriasis and eczema, and suitable treatment can then be suggested.

If dandruff or scalp symptoms are severe, there is now some good news for sufferers. A specific antifungal shampoo called Nizoral is available on prescription and is very effective. Your doctor may suggest using this twice weekly for about four weeks, interspersed with milder medicated shampoos on other days. You may then be advised to use the antifungal shampoo less frequently to prevent symptoms recurring. Regular hair-washing with this shampoo may also help if your eyelids are inflamed and crusty, although another organism – the staphylococcus – is often involved in this case too. It causes a condition known as blepharitis, to which many people are prone from childhood. Symptoms can usually be controlled by removing crusts from the eyelids by bathing them with a cotton wool bud dipped in baby shampoo, diluted to half strength, and then applying an antibiotic ointment to the rims.

Your doctor may prescribe antifungal and/or various anti-inflammatory applications for skin rashes on other parts of the body due to seborrhoeic dermatitis; taking antibiotics by mouth may be necessary if the rash becomes infected by other germs.

So, if the usual medicated shampoos do not keep your dandruff at bay, don't feel that it is too minor a problem to bother your doctor with. Any of these conditions can be very distressing and embarrassing and there is a lot that can now be done to treat them.

**What's Available?** Capasal Therapeutic Shampoo, Denorex, Genisol, Lenium, Polytar Liquid

**My Favourite**    Polytar

**Homoeopathic Remedies**    Graphite, Sepia

## DERMATITIS
See DRY SKIN CONDITIONS p.59

## DIARRHOEA
Diarrhoea is an extremely common symptom involving loose or liquid bowel movements and frequent or speedy trips to the loo. It is also often accompanied by cramping pain in the lower abdomen. It can make you feel quite exhausted and if you're on holiday it can ruin your fun.

Most attacks of diarrhoea are caused by gastro-intestinal infections – you can think of them as the body's way of getting rid of harmful substances. If more than one member of your family suffers at the same time, it is likely the diarrhoea was caused by something you've all eaten. If you have just come back from a trip away, you might have been exposed to standards of hygiene that do not match up to what you are used to, resulting in what we know as 'holiday tummy'. If your diarrhoea is accompanied by vomiting, food poisoning is also a likely cause. Gastric flu could be the culprit, too.

Another common cause of diarrhoea is stress. A job interview or a driving test can reduce the toughest of us to a bundle of nerves. Eating large amounts of food with laxative properties, such as prunes, can have an adverse effect. Diarrhoea can be a side-effect of taking certain drugs – antibiotics, for example. Tetracycline, a commonly prescribed antibiotic, can destroy friendly bacteria which normally live in the bowel and are part of our natural defences against more harmful bacteria. Consequently, if they are destroyed, the harmful ones – perhaps resistant to the antibiotic – can thrive. But if this happens to you, don't just stop taking the antibiotics. Ring your doctor and ask for advice.

Whatever the cause, most attacks of diarrhoea usually clear up quickly and without medical attention. The best way to treat yourself is not eating for 24 hours and drinking plenty of watery drinks. Frequent bursts of diarrhoea can make you feel even more ill as your body becomes dehydrated. The greatest risk from diarrhoea, and from vomiting too, is that the body's essential minerals are lost at the same time. Mineral depletion of this nature can make you feel weak and eventually faint. In a healthy person, water is essential to maintain normal body functions. Its importance is underlined by the fact that around half our body weight is water. Normally our kidneys balance the water lost in the urine and through perspiration against our fluid intake – we feel more thirsty and therefore drink more in hot weather, for instance.

Diarrhoea or sickness causes excessive loss of fluid, but if we are feeling ill, we may not feel thirsty. This means that our water balance is upset and we will continue to feel unwell until the fluid balance is restored.

To prevent mineral loss and dehydration you can buy ready-prepared sachets to be mixed with water, which are a combination of essential salts, minerals and energy-giving glucose. (This is known as oral rehydration therapy.) When these are mixed with the correct quantity of water as instructed, they are just the right strength for quick absorption, even by an inflamed stomach.

Medicines used to treat diarrhoea include powders which form a bulky mass inside the bowel to help carry away irritant substances. Typical examples are aluminium silicate (kaolin), calcium carbonate (chalk) and pectin (a purified carbohydrate product made from citrus fruits). Preparations made with these powders contain particles that swell up as they absorb water from the large intestine. This makes the faeces firmer and less runny. It's thought that these powders may absorb irritants and harmful chemicals along with the excess water.

Other drugs act on the muscular bowel wall to slow down bowel movements, relieving the familiar griping pains caused by diarrhoea. Typical examples are drugs from the opium family like codeine phosphate or morphine, which is usually mixed with kaolin.

In normally healthy adults, diarrhoea is rarely a serious condition – children and the elderly may suffer much more. This is because they are more sensitive to the problems of dehydration and often have less body fluid to lose. Babies under six months old are at the greatest risk from dehydration – their metabolic rate is high, their kidneys don't yet retain water very efficiently and they lose a greater proportion of water compared to their weight than adults do.

But even if you're a healthy adult, you should always consult your doctor if the condition doesn't improve within 48 hours, if the faeces contain blood, if there is severe abdominal pain or vomiting, or if you've just returned from a foreign country.

To help avoid gyppy tummy and the holiday runs – or worse – be careful with the ice in those long, cool drinks. Researchers writing in the *British Food Journal* pointed out some time ago that in Central America, four harmful germs were shown to survive even when frozen for 24 hours – and were still flourishing when melted in 86% proof tequila!

In the UK, hygiene standards can sometimes be inadequate when ice-making machines are sited in dirty, poorly ventilated areas, like cellars, and are not cleaned or serviced regularly. Ice is often put into the glass with the server's fingers and, in one survey, only half the ice-buckets were found to have lids – so dust and germs could float in. The researchers found germ contamination in ice-making machines as well as ice-buckets at the bar. More than one in two samples in the survey contained germs – and a large proportion of those were of the kind that could occur if someone didn't wash their hands after using the loo.

So, in future, when you are being careful about the cleanliness of your food and drink on holiday, beware of the humble ice cube. If the only available restaurant or bar doesn't look too clean, stick to the contents of mass-produced bottled drinks and thoroughly cooked food.

**What's Available**   Arret, Adult Kao-C and Junior Kao-C, Gluco-Lyte, Imodium, Opazimes, Rapolyte

**My Favourite**   Arret

# DRY SKIN CONDITIONS – ECZEMA, DERMATITIS AND PSORIASIS

Eczema and dermatitis are used as virtually interchangeable terms and generally mean inflammation of the skin. The main symptoms are itching and redness, accompanied by small blisters which often weep and form a crust. Eczema can take the form of small red patches on the limbs, or it can afflict large areas of the body. Although it is not usually a 'serious' disease, nor a contagious one, it can be severe, uncomfortable and unsightly, causing the sufferer to become exceptionally self-conscious. If you think you have eczema, see your doctor – although it is often hard to define the cause of eczema or to cure it completely, there are a number of treatments available to control it.

You can help combat the dryness, itching and flaking by preserving the moisture content of your skin. Avoid harsh or highly perfumed soaps or bath additives; instead, try using the emollient (moisturising) soaps, creams and specially made bath oils listed below, and when bathing use warm water instead of hot. These emollient products can be helpful when the skin becomes generally dry – often one of the minor complaints of pregnancy. Moisturising bath oils can make the surface of the bath slippery, so do be careful getting in and out.

Dry skin conditions can be a problem in childhood. About one child in ten suffers from infantile or atopic eczema. The symptoms are similar to those described above, but may look worse as a result of the child's scratching. Consult your doctor for treatment and advice. At home, keep the child's skin away from direct contact with wool or other rough fabrics – choose soft, pure cotton instead. Keep the child's fingernails short and use only gentle cleansing products suitable for infants.

Another form of skin complaint is known as contact dermatitis. This has similar symptoms to eczema but is specifically caused by contact with substances to which your skin is sensitive – household detergents or costume jewellery, for example. Protect your hands when using household cleansing fluids or chemicals, etc., and avoid contact with metals, dyes or even washing powders which may cause you problems. If you're not sure of the cause, consult your doctor, who may choose to carry out allergy tests. A mild hydrocortisone cream will ease discomfort by reducing inflammation and calming irritated skin.

Psoriasis can vary in severity from being a mild nuisance to, rarely, being so severe that the sufferer has to be admitted to hospital. With psoriasis, the skin cells grow much faster than usual. The skin cells divide and shed, which they normally do in any case (see DANDRUFF, p.53), but in just three to four days instead of the normal 25–28.

The precise cause isn't clear. What is known is that psoriasis can be triggered by stress, some drugs (beta-blockers given for high blood pressure, for example) and even an infection with a virus, such as German measles. Raised red patches with thick, silvery white scales appear on the skin, usually on the knees, elbows and scalp. On the scalp it's most noticeable as a thick white encrustation around the hairline and ears.

Psoriasis seems to be linked to heredity and can appear at any age, though it most commonly attacks those in their teens or twenties, affecting men and women equally. It can be a difficult condition to treat and unfortunately there's no long-term cure. Outbreaks tend to come and go – frequency and extent vary between individuals and cannot be predicted accurately.

Although psoriasis is not often harmful to the general

health and is not catching, the appearance of the skin can cause the sufferer great embarrassment and discomfort, especially when large areas are involved. The condition normally improves in the summer and gets worse again in the winter, but patches will sometimes clear up completely for years. On a day to day basis, emollient baths and creams (E45 for example) rubbed into the scaly patches can help to soothe the itching and flaking. Yoga, meditation and methods of relaxation – including holidays, especially in the sun, which is extremely beneficial for psoriasis – can all bring relief and, by encouraging a calmer outlook, may help prevent further flare-ups.

Sufferers can also benefit from eating more fish, especially oily fish like mackerel and herring. It's been suggested that one of the unsaturated fats in fish oils, EPA, is able to replace, within the body, another unsaturated fat, arachidonic acid. It is the metabolism – the body's usage – of this last acid which seems to be upset in someone who suffers from psoriasis (see VITAMINS p.213).

But despite all these possible remedies, active outbreaks should always be seen by a doctor. If the psoriasis is widespread or persistent, specialised hospital treatments will be recommended.

**What's Available?**   Bath E45, Cream E45, Dermacort, Dermidex, Emulsiderm Medicaid (an antiseptic cream for tender skin areas), Lanacane, Lanacort, Oilatum Emollient, Oilatum Soap, Probase 3, Sudocrem, Wash E45

For contact dermatitis – HC45 Hydrocortisone Cream, Dermidex

**My Favourite**   Cream E45

**Homoeopathic Remedies**   Graphites, Rhus. Tox., Sulphur, Nelsons Graphites Cream (for dermatitis)

**Herbal Remedies**   Nelsons Calendula Cream (for sore and rough skin), Nelsons Evening Primrose Cream

# EAR WAX

Everyone has a certain amount of wax in their ears – it is a natural substance secreted by tiny glands in the skin of the ear similar to sweat glands. It helps protect the sensitive lining in the outer channel of the ear from infection and keeps it free of dust and flakes of skin. And just as some people sweat more than others, some people naturally produce more ear wax.

Usually the wax steadily crumbles away and is expelled from the ear as tiny flakes, to be replaced by a fresh supply of wax from within the ear. It only becomes troublesome when there is a build-up of too much wax which, if left for a long time, may harden or slip against the drum and cause hearing problems.

When you first become aware of the familiar slight 'muzziness' caused by a build-up of wax, try softening the wax with a little olive oil at body temperature dropped into the ear(s) two or three times a day. Alternatively, there are special ear-wax softening drops, sometimes medicated, which your pharmacist can recommend. The wax may then gradually slide out on its own.

However, I must urge you to take great care with your ears – never delve inside too deeply or you could damage the drum. Do not attempt to clean or unblock your ears with cotton wool buds, nor use force or instruments in the ear. And never use ear drops to soften wax if your ears are inflamed or infected.

If you do use drops and after two or three days your ears still don't feel clear, consult your doctor – your ears may need syringing with warm water.

**What's Available?**    Cerumol, Cupal Wax Aid, Earex, Exterol Ear Drops

**My Favourite**    Cerumol

# ECZEMA

See DRY SKIN CONDITIONS p.59

# FEVER

A fever, the result of a high temperature (over 38°C/100.4°F) which makes you sweat or shiver, can be a symptom of any one of several illnesses, but is usually a sign that your body is fighting infection. Coughs, colds and other infections are often accompanied by aches, pains and feverishness.

To help reduce a fever, take the recommended dose of aspirin, ibuprofen or paracetamol – paracetamol for children (see PAINKILLERS p.89 for products containing these ingredients). Drink plenty of cold, alcohol-free fluids. Sponging the body with tepid water can be helpful in cases of high fever – but when the temperature is as high as 40°C/103°F, at least phone your doctor for advice.

**What's Available?**   For children: Calpol Infant Suspension, Calpol Six Plus, Cupanol Under 6, Cupanol Over 6, Fenning's Children's Cooling Powders, Medised, Junior Paraclear, Panadol Junior and Baby/Infant Elixir

For adults: see PAINKILLERS p.89 for list of products containing aspirin, ibuprofen or paracetamol

**My Favourite**   For children: Calpol Infant Suspension or Calpol Six Plus

# FIBROSITIS
See RHEUMATIC PAIN p.100

# GUM DISEASE – GINGIVITIS, BLEEDING GUMS

Let's start with the good news – our dental health has improved enormously over the last twenty years and continues to do so. Nevertheless, periodontal (gum) disease is still the commonest of all diseases in the world, not just in Britain, and up to one in five adults in this country will have lost all their teeth by the time they are sixty, mainly because of this condition.

Gum disease can appear as an inflammation of the gum margins (the gingival margins). Gunge – a mixture of bacteria and food debris – collects in this crevice. Initially this may cause very mild inflammation, but sometimes it will inflame the gums sufficiently to make them sore and swollen – a condition called gingivitis. More seriously, the infection can spread beneath the gums and affect the deeper tissues which attach the tooth to the jaw-bone. It is then known as periodontitis or pyorrhoea and if it goes undetected and untreated the gums gradually recede, the bone becomes eroded and the teeth loosen and eventually fall out. Fortunately, gum disease can nearly always be prevented by good dental care and if you visit your dentist regularly, he or she will spot warning signs such as 'pocketing' – a gap developing between the teeth and gums. This can be measured and advice or treatment can then be given to halt the process.

Even the severest form of gum disease can be almost symptomless and surprisingly pain free, but one of the first signs that all is not well with your gums is if they look 'spongy' and inflamed, and bleed when you brush your teeth. Nearly everyone will experience this mild form of gingivitis from time to time and it is important to treat it promptly before it becomes more serious. Often a little extra care with your teeth-cleaning routine will do the trick.

The main cause of gum problems and tooth decay is plaque. This is a thin, colourless, sticky substance, composed mainly of bacteria, which forms almost continuously around the teeth and gum margins. If not removed by regular brushing it can build up and harden into a deposit known as tartar or calculus, which attracts further plaque. Tartar, unlike plaque, can be felt with the tongue and can only be removed by a dentist or dental hygienist using special instruments to scale the teeth.

When tartar has built up, every chew and every incorrect brushing can push the tender gums against the sandpaper-like plaque, making them bleed; more harmfully, it makes them shrink back, exposing more of the tooth. Indeed, many middle-aged and elderly people who have suffered from this process for years are said to be 'long in the tooth'. But this need not happen at all.

Food – particularly sugary and starchy food – interacts with plaque on the teeth and produces acid which eats away at the enamel. This acid attack can last anything from 40 minutes up to two hours after a meal or snack, so the number of times you eat during the day is important, as well as what you eat. If you must eat sweet things, try to limit them to meal times, when the other foods being eaten will 'dilute' the acid produced.

Eating a small piece of hard cheese at the end of a meal will help to neutralise the acid, as well as providing protective calcium. Contrary to popular belief, fruit such as apples do not clean the teeth and may only produce more acid. If you can, you should also avoid eating anything shortly before bedtime – our flow of saliva decreases when we sleep and its beneficial cleansing effects will therefore be less.

Saliva has another advantage – it contains a substance which neutralises acid. A recent study has shown that the Americans may have known a thing or two all along – chewing gum for a minimum of 20 minutes after a meal or snack increases the flow of saliva considerably, reducing the time that teeth are attacked by acid from two hours to just 20 minutes. Most people could benefit from it, including anyone who suffers from a dry mouth through taking certain medicines which can have the side-effect of drying up secretions. Any long-standing lack of saliva increases the likelihood of tooth decay, gum disease and mouth infections.

Of course, regular brushing – ideally for at least three minutes after breakfast and at bedtime – is also very important in keeping teeth and gums healthy. So too is the right toothbrush, replaced every three months. Ask your dental hygienist to advise you and show you the most effective way to clean your teeth. He or she will also show you how to use dental floss, useful for removing plaque from awkward crevices between the teeth and particularly necessary if your gums become inflamed and start to bleed.

Special 'disclosing tablets' which you chew and rinse around your teeth are helpful because they stain the plaque pink and enable you to see any you may have missed. Fluoride toothpaste strengthens the enamel and some toothpastes also contain an ingredient which reduces the build-up of tartar; there is also a fluoride toothpaste called Oral-B Zendium, which contains natural enzymes to help boost the mouth's defences against plaque. Antibacterial mouthwashes are available for treating mild gingivitis.

When electric toothbrushes were first invented, I thought they were the latest useless piece of 20th century equipment. How wrong I was! They vibrate electrically while the user is able to hold the small-headed brush at just the right angle. The result is the best cleaning job you can get without visiting your dental surgeon or hygienist. I never go anywhere without mine.

**What's Available?**   Bocasan Mouthwash, Dettol Mouthwash, Merocet, Oraldene

**My Favourite**   Oraldene

## HALITOSIS
See BAD BREATH p.22

## HAY FEVER
Hay fever is an allergic reaction which occurs in people who are particularly sensitive to pollen or spores released into the air by trees, grasses or moulds. Its medical name is seasonal allergic rhinitis and it is one of the most common allergies known. It is estimated that between 6 and 12 million people suffer – most between the ages of 10 and 40, with about one in six teenagers affected. It is also estimated that four million

working days are lost during June and July alone through hay fever.

Hay fever strictly refers to an allergy to grass pollen, but the term is often used to cover allergy to pollen from plants, shrubs and trees. Pollens released in spring are usually from trees, whilst in the summer flower, grass or weed pollens are released. In the autumn the symptoms are usually caused by pollen from autumn-flowering plants and the spores of some fungi. The sufferer's body reacts to pollen as though it were a dangerous threat like a germ, and does all it can to get rid of it by releasing a chemical called histamine. Histamine causes inflammation and irritation of the mucous membranes of the eyes, nose and ear passages. The eyes then water in an effort to wash away the pollen and the running nose and sneezing help eject pollen from the nose. Hay fever can also cause drowsiness.

Hay-fever sufferers are most at risk between May and September, when the 'pollen count' (the level of pollen in the air) is at its highest. So listen to the pollen count forecasts broadcast daily on television and local radio or check the weather reports in newspapers. A pollen count of 50 grains per cubic metre is enough to set most sufferers sneezing. The pollen count will be high on warm, dry and windy days because pollen released from grasses and trees is carried upwards by warm air. Also, warm, dry conditions are needed for pollen to be released in the first place.

Symptoms are often more severe in the morning, when pollen is released and carried upwards as the air temperature rises. They then become worse again in the evening as the temperature drops and the pollen grains drift back down.

There is no cure for hay fever, although steroid nasal sprays, available on prescription, are very helpful. But over-the-counter antihistamine tablets are one of the most popular forms of treatment. Antihistamines such as brompheniramine block the effects of histamine to stop the allergic reaction occurring and newer ones such as terfenadine produce little if any drowsiness. But care should be taken initially, as with all drugs taken for the first time, because there may be rare cases when the patient reacts badly.

For most relief, start taking antihistamines as soon as the first symptoms occur, although treatment can be started at any time. Nasal sprays containing decongestants which shrink swollen nasal tissues can provide relief from a blocked nose, but should only be used in the short term, since long-term use may actually aggravate the condition.

There are many self-help measures you can take to relieve the symptoms of hay fever. Wearing plain glasses or sunglasses can prevent much of the eye irritation, by stopping pollen grains entering the eyes. Avoid walking through grass or cutting it. Keep windows and doors closed, especially when lawns are being mowed. Stay away from pets if they have been outside. Try to plan your day to avoid being outdoors in the morning and evening when pollen counts are at their highest. Don't go on country walks and avoid parks or gardens on warm and sunny days, or, if this is impossible, wash your hair afterwards. Keep car windows and air vents closed when you're out driving. Don't smoke, because this causes further irritation to those susceptible to allergies.

A final word of hope. Most hay-fever sufferers do grow out of it eventually!

**What's Available?**    Aller-Eze, Aller-Eze Plus, Benylin Children's Cough Linctus, Congesteze, Contac 400, Dimotapp Elixir and Tablets, Dimotapp Elixir Paediatric, Dimotapp LA, Dristan, Fenox Nasal Drops, Flurex Inhalant, Hismanal, Otrivine Drops, Penetrol Catarrh Lozenges (for nasal congestion in hay fever), Penetrol Inhalant, Pollon-Eze, Resiston One, Seldane, Sinutab, Triominic, Triludan, Triludan Forte

**My Favourites**    Triludan, Aller-Eze

**Homoeopathic Treatments**    Nelsons Hay Fever Tablets

**Herbal Remedies**   Herbelix Specific

# HEADACHE

Headaches are an extremely common complaint, afflicting one person in three at least once a year, though some people do tend to suffer more than others. In fact, although we tend to use the word headache to describe any pain in the head, there are probably more than 100 different types of headache and they vary in intensity and location. Some develop gradually and clear up after an hour or two or a walk in the fresh air. Others can be extremely severe and can last more than 24 hours.

Two of the commonest types of headache are migraine, a severe, recurring headache which merits its own entry in this book (see p.79) and tension headache, sometimes known as muscle contraction headache.

With migraine, the pain is usually one sided and can be accompanied by other symptoms such as loss of appetite, nausea or vomiting. In a tension headache, the whole head throbs and feels as though there's a weight on top of it or a tight band around it. The pain is usually dull and persistent, originating in the muscles of the scalp. The tension headache is the most common symptom presented to a general practitioner and no one knows the cause, or why some people get a headache when they are emotionally upset and some don't.

Different sorts of headaches can also be brought on by other factors – drinking too much alcohol, sinusitis (see p.102), anxiety or being in an overheated room or smoky atmosphere are all common triggers. They may be the result of muscle strain in your neck, especially if the headache comes on after you have been reading or doing close work like sewing – you can become tense from concentrating for too long or from sitting in an awkward position.

For most minor headaches, it is worth trying the following self-help measures. Take the recommended dose of a mild painkiller such as aspirin or paracetamol (see PAIN-KILLERS p.89 for products containing these ingredients) – for best results, take the painkiller as soon as you feel the headache coming on. Drink plenty of water or other non-alcoholic, clear drinks. Rest in a quiet, darkened room may also be soothing and a warm bath will sometimes relieve tension.

Fortunately, most headaches are not a sign of serious disease, but if your headache is particularly severe; if it's accompanied by misty or blurred vision, nausea or vomiting; if there's no satisfactory explanation for a headache that is continuous or getting worse after three days, or comes back several times in the course of a week; or if you have injured your head during the past few days, you should consult your doctor for advice.

**What's Available?**    See PAINKILLERS p.89

**Homoeopathic Remedies**    Belladonna, Ignatia, Nat. Mur.

## HEAD LICE

Head lice are tiny brown insects with six short, stubbly legs. They're about the size of a pin head and live on human heads, laying six to eight pearly white coloured eggs a day (commonly known as nits). The eggs are attached near the base of the hair shaft – a favourite spot is around the ears. Each louse takes two weeks to mature and lives for 20 to 30 days if undetected. The lice feed on blood, using their specially developed mouth-parts to pierce the scalp. They even inject a local anaesthetic into the scalp to prevent their host feeling any pain, and an anticoagulant to stop the blood clotting, thus making it easier for them to feed! They can eventually make your head feel very itchy because, after about 10,000 bites, your immune system becomes under-standably irritated.

To check whether someone has head lice, dampen the hair and then bend the head over a plain sheet of paper.

Comb the hair thoroughly to see whether any insects drop out. Quickly part the hair to look out for moving lice. A magnifying glass will help.

Head lice can sometimes be a problem among schoolchildren. That's because the head louse has never had it so good. We and our children are healthier and cleaner than we have ever been, and the head louse loves it. Clean, healthy heads provide it with the perfect environment for perpetuating its lifestyle. Every time a clean-headed child comes into contact with another child's head as they play, the head louse moves from one head to another. Head lice can't jump or fly, nor do they live in bedding, furniture or clothes. The *only* way they can be passed on is by close head contact – a single louse can visit several heads in one day just by walking from one to another.

So if you or your children have head lice, please don't worry or feel ashamed. More than a million people a year in the UK get head lice, so there's no point in being embarrassed about it. It's also pretty well impossible to prevent children catching head lice from each other, as it's nothing to do with them being dirty or neglected. Like measles, mumps and chicken pox, it's just another of those things children are likely to catch once they start mixing with others.

If you have to deal with head lice, take the advice of your school nurse, pharmacist or health visitor, and use the lotions or shampoos they recommend. When applying a shampoo or lotion, remember to ensure that no part of the scalp is left uncovered; pay particular attention to the nape of the neck and behind the ears.

There are three main insecticides in use that kill head lice and their eggs – carbaryl, phenothrin and malathion. They are all equally effective if used according to the directions. But health authorities change their recommendations for louse treatment preparations every two to three years to prevent the lice building up a resistance to them. Your pharmacist can tell you what is currently in use in your area.

Bear in mind, too, that should a member of your family need treatment, you must treat the whole family – parents, grandparents, even lodgers – and then check them once a week to ensure they're still clear. Make sure your children's friends don't have lice either or there could be a risk of re-infection. It's wise – if not essential – to inform your child's school if you discover head lice.

Then after treatment, encourage all your family to comb their hair thoroughly every day, since the female louse – and there are many more of them than the male – must cling on to two hairs to survive; as combing or brushing separates the hair, the louse will then die. Once dead, it falls off harmlessly.

**What's Available?**   Carylderm Derbac Shampoo, Full Marks Shampoo, Lyclear, Prioderm, Suleo-C Carbaryl Shampoo, Suleo-C Carbaryl Lotion, Suleo-M Malathion Lotion

**My Favourites**   Carylderm, Lyclear

## HEARTBURN
See INDIGESTION AND HEARTBURN p.72

## HIVES
See URTICARIA p.117

## INDIGESTION AND HEARTBURN
Symptoms of indigestion, usually felt just below or behind the breast bone, vary from an uncomfortable feeling of fullness to nausea, pain, belching, heartburn and wind. Most people will suffer from indigestion from time to time. Often there is no recognisable pattern to the symptoms, but they may be noticeably worse just before or after a meal. Nearly one person in ten takes a remedy for some form of indigestion every day and of these one in three will have had symptoms for ten years or more. Three out of four

sufferers never consult a doctor. The problem becomes more common after middle age, particularly in those who are overweight. Sensitive, anxious people are also more prone to indigestion, as anxiety increases the output of acid secretions in the stomach.

The most common form of indigestion is called heartburn, an apt name as it well describes the symptoms – waves of burning pain behind the breast bone and sometimes a burning feeling in the throat. The pain can be mistaken for heart pain (angina), but in fact angina improves with rest, whereas heartburn is usually worse when the sufferer is lying down. It is easy to see why when we look more closely at what causes it.

The stomach produces strong acid secretions which help to digest and sterilise our food. The stomach lining has a mucous coating which protects it against the acid, but the oesophagus – the gullet down which food passes from the mouth to the stomach – does not. Normally a ring of muscle – the cardiac sphincter – at the bottom end of the oesophagus acts like a trapdoor and prevents acid rising up from the stomach. Sometimes, however – if the muscle becomes a little lax, for instance, as it often does during pregnancy – small amounts of acid will enter the lower part of the oesophagus – a process known as reflux. It is normal for this to happen occasionally and the saliva we are constantly swallowing will usually be enough to neutralise the acid without symptoms being caused. Also, contractions of the muscle walls of the gullet prevent the acid rising by keeping food and saliva moving downwards.

However, if reflux occurs too often, the oesophagus will gradually become inflamed and painful as the acid burns into the tissues. This inflammation is called oesophagitis. Without effective treatment the lining of the gullet can eventually become ulcerated and constricted by scarring so that swallowing food can be difficult. Other changes in the cells may also develop in time. It is important, therefore, to treat heartburn early on to prevent oesophagitis progressing.

Indigestion can have other causes – secretions such as pepsin (an enzyme which aids digestion) and bile from the liver (which helps digest fatty foods) are also capable of irritating the vulnerable stomach. Anxious people will often, unconsciously, swallow more air with their food and eat faster than others, causing distention, a rumbling stomach and belching. This type of indigestion may be relieved by learning techniques for relaxation (with the help of cassettes, for instance) and by eating smaller, more frequent meals, slowly.

Many people think that eating greasy, rich or spicy foods, or eating too much too quickly, are the main causes of heartburn. In fact, although these do play a part, smoking more than ten cigarettes a day and drinking heavily are the most common causes, as both of these relax the cardiac sphincter and therefore make reflux more likely. Bouts of indigestion are therefore sometimes a warning signal that the body is being abused – alcohol, especially on an empty stomach, and smoking both stimulate acid production and inflame the stomach.

Some drugs – antibiotics, iron tablets and aspirin, for example – can also inflame the oesophagus and cause heartburn, especially if they are taken with too little fluid or just before going to bed. Citrus fruits, chocolate, coffee and, perhaps surprisingly, peppermint are other possible culprits. Heartburn is also a common symptom of a hiatus hernia, whereby part of the stomach protrudes upwards at the point where the oesophagus passes through a gap in the diaphragm. A sensitivity to certain foods, such as sugar and milk, can also cause unpleasant indigestion, as can fatty foods for some people. Cutting down on stimulants and avoiding foods found to aggravate the symptoms will, in this case, usually relieve them.

Indigestion and heartburn are, of course, also common during pregnancy. Being overweight, large meals and lack of exercise are other predisposing factors. If indigestion or heartburn is worrying or persistent, a doctor's examination and perhaps some special investigations may be necessary to exclude underlying causes such as hiatus hernia, peptic ulcer or gall bladder trouble.

When no such cause can be found, and in most cases of occasional indigestion, self-help measures can help. Don't smoke or drink too much alcohol, coffee or acidic fruit drinks. Lose weight if necessary. It's better to eat several small meals a day rather than one large one and to avoid eating just before going to bed. Eat slowly, sitting upright – not slouched in front of the television – and chew your food thoroughly before swallowing. Get used to bending down from the knees rather than from the waist and avoid stooping after meals. Don't wear tight belts or corsets, as they increase pressure on the stomach.

If heartburn is troublesome at night, raise the head end of the bed about eight inches – two standard house bricks are about the right height. This helps to keep the acid down in the stomach and is much more effective than using extra pillows, because you will probably slide off these in your sleep. A glass of milk before bedtime helps, too.

Combined with these measures, a regular dose, in between meals, of an antacid medicine bought from the chemist should be all that is needed to ease indigestion. These medicines neutralise stomach acid, help prevent inflammation and relieve pain. Around £42 million were spent on indigestion remedies in the UK in 1990 and as you can imagine there are several different types – for example, aluminium hydroxide, calcium carbonate, magnesium hydroxide and sodium bicarbonate. Antacids can be combined with substances called alginates, which float on the contents of the stomach and stop the gastric juices splashing upwards (refluxing) and irritating the gullet, or with drugs to disperse wind.

Some antacids are more effective than others. Magnesium hydroxide can take a while to have any effect but relief is fairly long lasting. Some remedies – those containing calcium, for instance – wear off quickly, and by over-neutralising the existing acid in the stomach, may have the rebound effect of actually stimulating further acid production. Also, the calcium and sodium salts contained in some antacid medicines will be absorbed into the bloodstream, and this is undesirable in the longer term.

Remember that all antacids can interfere with the absorption of other drugs, so check with your pharmacist if you are taking any other medicines. You will probably find that a particular brand of antacid will work better than others for your indigestion, so it will often be a case of trial and error.

**What's Available?**    Actal, Alka-Seltzer (for headache with upset stomach), Andrews Liver Salt, Andrews Answer (for headache with upset stomach), Andursil Tablets and Liquid, Asilone Tablets, Aludrox Tablets and Liquid, Bismag, Bisodol Powder and Tablets, Bisodol Extra, Dijex, Gastrils Antacid Pastilles, Gaviscon, Gelusil Tablets, Indigestion Lozenges, Lanes Charcoal Tablets, Milk of Magnesia, Morland, Premiums, Rennie, Rennie Gold, Rennie Plus

**My Favourites**    Rennie, Actal

**Homoeopathic Remedies**    Carbo. Veg., Kali. Phos., Nux. Vom.

## INFLUENZA

People often say they have flu when really they have some other virus which is giving them 'flu-like' symptoms – and so-called 'gastric flu' is certainly not due to the influenza virus. But for many people the symptoms of flu – a dreadfully ill feeling, sometimes with acutely painful muscles, a high temperature and a headache – are such that the sufferer may suspect he or she has been afflicted with a very serious illness.

There are three main types of 'proper' flu virus recognisable under a microscope – A, B and C, the C variety being mild and insignificant. The A type is highly infectious and often develops into a widespread epidemic or even a worldwide pandemic – the 'Asian flu' of 1957 and the 'Hong Kong flu' of 1968 were caused by the A flu virus. Influenza

B spreads less rapidly, tends to remain localised to communities or institutions such as schools and colleges and to occur at intervals of about four years.

Flu is caught by breathing in the virus through germs in the air breathed out by sufferers. The virus then attacks and inflames the lining of the nose, throat and air passages, causing symptoms similar to those of a severe cold. Joint and muscle aches and pains, headache and fever are also common, as the virus is carried by the bloodstream to other parts of the body. The worst is usually over in about a week, though an attack of flu can leave the sufferer feeling tired and depressed for some time afterwards. The very young or very old and those with chronic chest or heart problems, kidney disease or diabetes are particularly vulnerable to the more severe effects of flu and, because of the way it is spread, are more likely to catch it if living in an institution.

Although antibiotics will have no effect on the virus itself (or indeed on viruses in general), your doctor will often prescribe an antibiotic at the first sign of flu for anyone with a 'weak chest' – chronic bronchitis sufferers, for example – to prevent a secondary bacterial infection developing and causing more damage. Coughing up green or yellow sputum is an indication of this type of infection and means you should consult your doctor, as antibiotics may be necessary.

Otherwise, rest in bed, take two aspirin or paracetamol every four hours, or follow the instructions for taking your preferred painkiller (see PAINKILLERS p.89). Children with flu are not generally recommended to take aspirin, however. Drink plenty of liquid. Steam inhalations can make breathing easier and linctus should relieve any cough you may have (see COUGHS p.45 for product information). To relieve flu symptoms such as blocked sinuses, stuffed-up nose and catarrh, refer to what's available for a common cold (p.33). For feverishness in children as part of flu, see FEVER p.63. But the body's own defences – the antibodies we produce in response to infection – should do the rest.

With most viruses – measles for instance – the antibodies

we develop after one attack give us a natural, lasting immunity. In other cases, a specific vaccine can protect us by stimulating effective antibodies. This is because the virus does not change. Not so with flu. The vaccine produced against flu has to be updated annually because the virus itself alters and keeps developing slightly different strains. So, although the antibodies we produced if we caught flu last year will give us resistance to some attacks in future, they will not protect us against the new strains that may have developed since. Vaccine manufacturers must keep adding to their anti-flu 'cocktail' and try to keep pace.

Immunisation against flu is becoming increasingly widespread in Britain. A vaccination given in the autumn provides about 70% protection and lasts about a year. Most doctors believe it's worthwhile for the vulnerable groups – it's estimated that several thousand people die in the UK every year from the effects of flu and around eight out of every ten of those are over the age of 65.

Anyone at special risk should consult his or her doctor for advice. The risk categories include anyone who suffers from chronic chest, heart or kidney disease or diabetes. The vaccine should also benefit elderly people or children living together – in residential homes or schools, for example. Other groups at risk include those who have conditions such as AIDS which affect the body's immune system, or those who are taking drugs that are known to dampen the natural defences.

Do I have a flu injection myself, you may ask? No, but then I'm not in the high risk category and there's little evidence that the fit population suffer too much overall disadvantage from contact with the real flu germ. We may suffer some unpleasant symptoms, but they are quite often mild, and the protection the real virus germs provoke in our bodies is stronger and more lasting than that provided by vaccination – although, as I said, the variation between the different strains of flu virus means that neither natural immunisation nor vaccination lasts forever. And do high doses of Vitamin C give you protection? Again, the answer is unclear. You pays your money or you takes your chance, and I prefer to take my chance!

There isn't really anything you can do to prevent yourself getting a cold or flu. But when you do have a bout of flu, it is foolish and unfair to others to struggle to work, unless your presence is absolutely essential – you are almost certain to infect someone else. Rest is a natural aid to recovery, so by staying quietly at home you will be doing yourself a favour, too. If everyone, at the very first sign of flu, became a recluse for a few days, epidemics and pandemics would probably become a thing of the past!

**What's Available**   Catarrh-Ex. See also COLD (p.33), COUGHS (p.45), FEVER (p.63)

# INSOMNIA
See SLEEPLESSNESS p.105

# MIGRAINE
Anyone who's ever had a migraine – and you can include me in that – can understand the misery it brings. Yet migraine sufferers are often branded as 'neurotic' and made to feel guilty about their 'weakness'. This is completely unfair, as studies have shown that there is no typical 'migraine personality'. Migraine affects as many as one in ten people (mainly women) of any race, occupation, class or age, including children. More than half will have a relative – often their mother – with the same problem.

Frequency of attacks varies greatly, from only once or twice a year to several times a week. Severity and type of symptoms differ widely, too. A sufferer may find that he or she has a mild attack at one time and then a severe one next time. The severity is usually related to extra tension and strain and it is really very important to remain as calm as possible.

So what makes a migraine more than 'just a headache'? The pain is usually one sided, and in the 'common' type, there are other symptoms such as loss of appetite, nausea or vomiting. A few sufferers will have the 'classic' type of migraine, preceded, 20–30 minutes before the headache itself, by warning symptoms – called an aura – which may include flashing lights before the eyes, shimmering or double vision, slurred speech, numbness and giddiness. These symptoms are probably due to a sudden constriction in some of the blood vessels in the brain.

The headache comes on as these vessels then expand and the blood surges through, leading to the characteristic throbbing headache. Many experts believe that this constriction and dilation of the blood vessels is brought about by changing levels of certain chemicals circulating in the body, such as adrenaline – also released during stress – and prostaglandins. Adrenaline tenses the muscles, the heart and its blood vessels to prepare us for 'fight or flight'. Prostaglandins sensitise the nerve endings to make us more alert. In susceptible people, they will 'overdo' it and cause the above symptoms. Studies also suggest that there may be a slight difference – perhaps inherited – in the biochemical make-up of migraine sufferers which makes them more susceptible.

The trigger for an attack can be emotional or physical and common ones include anxiety, excitement, depression, changes in weather or routine, bending for long periods (such as when gardening), hot baths, loud noises, flashing or bright light, including that from a VDU screen. Glare filters are now available which many people find helpful. Alcohol, especially red wine, is one of the worst culprits, and certain foods, for example chocolate, cheese, fried foods, citrus fruit, onions, tea, coffee, wheat flour, pork and seafood, are other common triggers.

Irregular meals, dieting or a long lie-in can provoke a migraine, probably because of the drop in the body's blood sugar. Then a few biscuits or a sweet drink may be enough to stave off a full attack. It's extremely important to make sure you always eat properly and pay attention to your diet. If you think you'll have to go a long time without a proper meal, keep an emergency ration of a small snack of some sort with you.

Hormones can also play a part as far as women are concerned – some only have a migraine around the time of their menstrual period or if they are taking the contraceptive pill. Many find their migraines improve, or stop altogether, after the menopause.

To help you and your doctor pinpoint your special triggers, try to keep a diary, noting the day and time of your attacks, everything you eat and drink, meal times, daily activities, particular worries and, for women, the dates of your periods. If you think you are suffering from migraine or experience a migraine attack for the first time, consult your doctor for a proper diagnosis and advice on treatment. This will also reassure you that your migraines are not due to a tumour or to high blood pressure – two very common and usually quite unfounded fears.

Treatment will depend on the frequency of attacks and the apparent causes. Simply adjusting your habits may help considerably. Any medicines should be taken at the first sign of an attack, so always keep them handy. It usually helps to rest quietly in a darkened room in the early stages. During a migraine attack, the action of the gut slows down and painkillers may not be well absorbed. Some of the medicines available from your doctor speed up absorption as well as relieving the nausea and pain. Other drugs act by constricting the dilated blood vessels, but follow the instructions precisely as overuse can actually bring on a headache similar to migraine.

If migraine attacks are very frequent, your doctor may prescribe long-term preventive treatment, such as one of the drugs often used to control high blood pressure. Over the counter, you can buy painkillers (see p.89). Remember that migraine is different from other types of headache in that it's often accompanied or preceded by other symptoms already mentioned.

Anti-inflammatory medicines like aspirin and ibuprofen can prevent the release of prostaglandins and so are recommended for migraine – although paracetamol can help ease the pain of a headache, too. There are also tablets available over the counter which are especially designed to relieve a migraine headache. These can contain analgesics combined with buclizine hydrochloride or cyclizine hydrochloride – antihistamines to prevent vomiting and reduce nausea. Sufferers usually work out which treatment suits them best.

If stress or anxiety seems to be the underlying cause of your migraines, relaxation exercises or hypnotherapy may be helpful. And trying 'alternative' treatments like acupuncture is something I would recommend to anyone who has found no joy through traditional methods of coping with migraine.

You could not be blamed for wondering why acupuncture seems to have such a surprising success rate for so many completely different ailments and diseases. The reason is that it's not just some ancient superstition that's now available as a last resort. It works by triggering the brain to secrete its own chemicals, which function rather like natural painkillers or tranquillisers, so providing relief for sufferers.

Period-time migraines often respond to treatment with the hormone progesterone. Recent research has shown that a daily dose of a humble plant called feverfew (it looks like a miniature chrysanthemum and is now sold by many nursery gardens – the botanical name for the variety of feverfew you need is *Tanacetum parthenium*) helps many people to control their migraine. Two or three leaves can be eaten in a sandwich sweetened with a little honey, and feverfew capsules and tablets are available from some chemists and health-food shops.

**What's Available?**    Hom-Bidor 1% Tablets, Migraclear, Migraleve

**Homoeopathic Remedies**    Kali. Bich., Nat. Mur., Silicea

**Herbal Remedies**    Herbal Labs Feverfew 125, Golden Health Feverfew (English Grains)

# MOUTH ULCERS

Mouth ulcers tend to be small lesions on the tongue, on the inside of the cheeks or the roof of the mouth – and like so many minor problems, they are something that everybody will suffer from at some stage. They're often called aphthous ulcers and have a pale grey base and a slightly raised yellowish edge, tinged with a narrow, inflamed border.

Some people find ulcers hurt so unbearably that eating is impossible. Fortunately, for most they're just a temporary nuisance. They may be painful, even unsightly, but they are harmless and will disappear of their own accord after a week or so.

Despite all the research that has been carried out, we still have no real idea what causes mouth ulcers. We do know, however, that a person is more likely to develop them if he or she is under stress, unwell, over-tired, depressed or suffering from any form of emotional upset. People in high-powered jobs, young mothers and toddlers with flu all seem to be prone to attacks. Many women find they suffer from mouth ulcers almost monthly, around the time of their period.

If you have ever had a mouth ulcer, you will be able to recognise the symptoms. Hours before they appear, the mouth will become over-sensitive or you'll experience a burning or tingling sensation. Pretty soon, blisters with red margins appear in your mouth. When they erupt they produce small, round ulcers with greyish or dirty white centres, which are often extra sensitive to salty and acidic foods.

Mouth ulcers may clear up within a few days or take over a week to disappear. In most cases, no treatment is needed. But if the ulcer is particularly painful, an antiseptic mouthwash or pastilles or gel containing antiseptics and local anaesthetics can ease soreness. A supplement of folic acid, one of the B vitamins, may help shorten an attack or prevent another one occurring (see VITAMINS p.213).

Badly fitting dentures can rub against the side or roof of the mouth and sometimes this can cause an outbreak of ulcers. If that is the source of your problem, a cream called Aezodent, which is mildly anaesthetic and has a gum 'adhesive' to help hold the denture securely in place, may bring relief.

If any ulcer is abnormally large or lasts for more than two weeks, you should certainly consult your doctor. But if you find you're getting frequent attacks of ulcers, even though they heal quickly, it may well be worth taking a careful look at the way you live and trying to reduce any stress in your life. Find a method of regular relaxation that suits you and your lifestyle – that might mean taking a form of gentle exercise or listening quietly to music. Another simple way to combat stress is to try to get more sleep – a few early nights can work wonders.

**What's Available?**    Aezodent, Anbesol, Bioral Gel, Ress Q, Rinstead Adult Gel, Rinstead Pastilles, Ulc-Aid Gel, Ulc-Aid Lozenges

**My Favourites**    Rinstead Pastilles, Anbesol

## MUSCULAR ACHES, PAINS, SPRAINS AND STRAINS

As more and more people are heeding advice to take regular exercise, a few are bound to suffer a so-called soft tissue (as opposed to bone) injury at some time – strains, sprains or bruising, for example, to muscles, ligaments, tendons or the capsule (lining) of a joint. The elderly and those who have taken up or returned to a sport late in life are more at risk than the young and fit.

A strain is a slight tearing of a muscle or the tendon attaching it to a bone, usually caused by overstretching it, whereas a sprain is a tear in a joint capsule or its supportive ligaments, due to twisting or forcing the joint beyond its normal range of movement.

Other soft tissue problems include capsulitis (inflammation of a joint lining due to a twisting or jarring injury), bursitis (inflammation of the fluid-filled bursae that act as cushions at points of wear and tear) and epicondylitis (inflammation where muscle tendons join the bony points of the elbow). If pain and tenderness are on the outer point, epicondylitis is commonly known as tennis elbow, if on the inner side golfer's elbow, but any activity that overuses these tendons can cause the same symptoms – painting a ceiling or hammering, for example.

Another condition, often in the news these days, is tenosynovitis or repetitive strain injury (RSI) – painful inflammation of the tendon sheaths in the hands, wrists or arms, which can be very disabling. Typists, factory workers or anyone using repetitive movements for hours on end are particularly prone. Regular rest breaks and more varied work will help prevent RSI developing.

When a strain or sprain first occurs, chemicals are released into the damaged tissues – they include prostaglandins, which sensitise nerve endings and cause pain, inflammation and swelling. Treatment which prevents or cuts down the release of prostaglandins is therefore likely to be helpful. Medicines known as NSAIDs – non-steroid anti-inflammatory drugs – such as aspirin and ibuprofen, act in this way and the sooner they can be given after an injury the better (see PAINKILLERS p.89 for product list). Ibuprofen is also available as a cream from pharmacists and on prescription – its commercial name is Proflex or Ibuleve. Studies show that it relieves the pain and other symptoms when rubbed directly into the injured area, without the risk of side-effects, nausea for example, that tablets may cause.

Lasonil is another cream that can help soft tissue injuries – it contains heparinoid, an anti-inflammatory agent. There are also soothing rubs, gels and sprays available to help ease muscular aches and pains. Sometimes an anti-inflammatory injection – into the tender spot of a tennis elbow, for instance – will be advised if the pain is acute.

First-aid measures in the initial 48 hours after injury can be very helpful and speed recovery. Rest the injured part as much as possible and raise it to reduce swelling (support an injured arm in a sling, for example). An ice pack will reduce bruising and swelling and will also relieve pain; contrary to popular belief, a hot bath will make matters worse, because it speeds up the flow of blood and increases swelling. Wrap the ice in a wet cloth or flannel to protect the skin from iceburn and frostbite and apply the pack to the injured part for ten minutes every few hours. A compression bandage such as tubigrip, worn continuously for at least two days, will help, too, but watch for numbness, tingling or the skin colour changing to white or blue – signs that the bandage is too tight.

Ideally, try to prevent injury occurring in the first place. Exercise, though undoubtedly good for you, should not be overdone. If you are unaccustomed to it, expert tuition is often advisable and do take things gradually to begin with.

**What's Available?**   Fiery Jack Rubbing Ointment, Ibuleve, Lasonil, PR Spray, Proflex. See also PAINKILLERS p.89

**My Favourite**   PR Spray

## NAPPY RASH
All babies suffer from a red or sore bottom from time to time, however well you look after them. For the first couple of years or so of a child's life, the area of skin around his or her bottom is constantly in contact with – and so under attack from – urine and faeces. Nappy rash can take the form of just a few spots, or a more severe rash. It can be triggered by several factors, such as diarrhoea or rawness caused by urine that's irritating the skin inside a chafing nappy. Bacteria in the faeces can react with urine to produce ammonia – not very pleasant on tender, young skin. This type of contamination often encourages a fungus similar to the one that causes thrush.

To avoid nappy rash change your baby's nappy frequently and clean and dry his or her bottom and skin creases thoroughly. It's helpful to leave your baby without a nappy on as often as possible – air is a great benefit. Use a barrier cream – zinc and castor oil cream, for example, to protect the baby's skin from constant exposure to moisture. If you use terry towelling nappies, be careful to sterilise them properly as well as ensuring that they're well rinsed – traces of detergent can also be an irritant.

If the baby's bottom already shows signs of a rash, specially formulated nappy rash creams can soothe it, help fight infection or prevent moisture irritating the skin. If the rash doesn't seem to get any better after a week of this treatment, ask the advice of your doctor or health visitor.

**What's Available?** Conotrane, Daktarin Cream or Powder, Drapolene Cream, E45 Cream, Medicaid, Morhulin Cod-Liver Oil Ointment, Morsep, Savlon Nappy Rash Cream, Sudocrem

**My Favourites** Sudocrem, Drapolene

**Homoeopathic Remedies** Arsen. Alb., Calendula Cream

# NASAL CONGESTION
See SINUS PAIN, NASAL CONGESTION AND CATARRH p.102

# NETTLE RASH
See URTICARIA p.117

# NEURALGIA
Pain resulting from a nerve being over-stimulated, compressed or squeezed is known as neuralgia. It can be very uncomfortable as the pain isn't just felt at the point of stimulation or pressure, but can be experienced along the full course of the nerve. It is sometimes described as an intense pain similar to the most agonising toothache.

This often excruciating pain can be felt anywhere in the body, depending on which nerve is affected. A fractured bone, severe bruising around a bone or a 'slipped' disc can press on a nerve and cause neuralgia; so, too, can an infection like shingles. This causes a different kind of pain, since it's the nerve itself which is inflamed by the nerve-specific shingles infection.

You can treat yourself with mild painkillers (see p.89 for product list) or ask your doctor to prescribe stronger ones if the pain is severe. But if the shingles pain persists for longer than a month, you will need your doctor's prescribed medicine. This is because the shingles will have developed into PHN – post-herpetic neuralgia – which won't respond to the usual painkillers.

**What's Available?**   See PAINKILLERS p.89

## ORAL THRUSH

Denture wearers may be familiar with the problem of oral thrush as a result of chafing, although it can also affect babies, people suffering from diabetes, those who are generally unwell and not at their strongest, or those taking steroid or antibiotic drugs.

It's caused by a yeast-like fungus called *Candida albicans* which is also responsible for vaginal thrush. This usually lives harmlessly in the mouth and the intestines. Bacteria are normally able to keep it under control, but sometimes it will suddenly grow very rapidly, producing soreness and white flecks inside the mouth, painful cracks in the skin in the corners of the mouth and/or creamy yellow patches inside the mouth and throat.

If you think you or your baby have oral thrush, consult a doctor, who may prescribe an antifungal medicine or lozenges. Thrush will not go away without treatment. But if the patient is your baby, you can help by sterilising dummies frequently and, if you're breast-feeding, taking extra care with nipple hygiene.

If you have suffered from oral thrush before and have had the symptoms diagnosed by your doctor, you'll be interested to know that an oral gel formerly only available on prescription can now be obtained from chemists on a pharmacist's recommendation. Daktarin Oral Gel contains miconazole, an antifungal and antibacterial drug that kills the yeast cells. It can be effective in the treatment of fungal infections of the lips, mouth and throat – and that includes oral thrush in babies and adults and the kind that is due to denture chafing. It's sugar free, has a pleasant orange flavour and is specially formulated to stick to mucous membranes for up to six hours after application. For denture chafing, it may be useful to smear a small amount of Daktarin on to the denture plate. Relief from symptoms may occur quickly, but it's important that you continue to use Daktarin for up to two days after the symptoms have cleared. If you're pregnant you should consult your doctor before using the gel.

**What's Available?**   Daktarin Oral Gel, Oraldene

# PAINKILLERS

Painkillers, or analgesics, can be used to treat pain resulting from a wide variety of symptoms. They can ease pain in headaches, migraine, neuralgia, colds and influenza and help reduce temperature, rheumatic pain, period pain, dental pain, back ache, muscular pain and sore throats. So it's hardly surprising that analgesics take up the biggest share of the market in over-the-counter medicines. In 1990 alone £145 million was spent on them!

Consequently there's a vast range of analgesics on sale in shops, supermarkets and chemists in soluble or tablet form – soluble painkillers are said to work more quickly because the active ingredient is absorbed into the bloodstream faster than solid tablets.

Over-the-counter analgesics mainly contain aspirin,

paracetamol or a combination of the two, sometimes with the addition of the stimulant caffeine. Some also contain small quantities of codeine and others contain ibuprofen. If you are taking one kind of analgesic you should not take another within four hours – overdoses can be dangerous.

Aspirin – and its associated sodium salicylate compounds – is a non-narcotic (non-addictive) analgesic. It relieves pain, reduces fever and inflammation, and can improve the symptoms of arthritis. It's also thought to prevent blood clots from forming. It works by blocking the production of prostaglandins, which would pass pain signals on to the brain.

Aspirin can irritate the stomach and if it's used for a long time it can cause bleeding. That's why aspirin should be taken after food; if you must take it on an empty stomach, have a glass of milk at the same time. Avoid alcohol when you're taking aspirin, as it adds to the chances of the stomach being irritated. Do not take aspirin if you have a stomach ulcer. It is not usually recommended near the end of a pregnancy, either.

There also appears to be some connection between young children taking aspirin and developing Reye's Syndrome – a rare condition, affecting only about seven children in a million, which causes brain inflammation and liver damage. It is not even certain that aspirin is implicated in this condition, but the possibility is enough to make doctors feel that children under 12 should not generally be given aspirin. Paracetamol is a safe alternative.

Paracetamol is also a non-narcotic analgesic. It's gentler on the stomach than aspirin and won't cause bleeding. But large doses can cause serious damage to the liver and kidneys. It can be used during pregnancy, but always check with your doctor if you think you need to take it for more than an occasional dose.

Paracetamol works in a similar way to aspirin, but, unlike aspirin, it only blocks prostaglandin production in the brain, rather than elsewhere in the body as well. This means that it does not reduce inflammation, as aspirin does. For children it is available in a specially formulated suspension form – in the Calpol range, for example.

Ibuprofen is an NSAID (non-steroidal anti-inflammatory drug) which relieves pain, reduces inflammation and lowers temperature. It has been found in use to be gentler on the stomach than aspirin (though there is no obvious explanation for this as they work in similar ways) and as a result is as well tolerated as paracetamol. However, as with other pain-relievers, it shouldn't be taken if you have a stomach ulcer or other stomach disorder. Asthma sufferers and anyone who is allergic to aspirin should only take ibuprofen after consulting their doctor. It's not usually prescribed for pregnant women.

Codeine is a mild narcotic (habit-forming) drug which is mainly used in over-the-counter analgesics in combination with paracetamol, or paracetamol and aspirin in the case of Veganin. It blocks transmission of pain signals within the brain and the spinal cord, but used on its own does not have much painkilling effect. While its use in combination as mentioned above has always been popular, the benefits of this over the use of aspirin or paracetamol on their own are open to doubt. Do not take codeine-containing medicines if you are pregnant, or think you may be, as it has not been tested to prove that it is safe during pregnancy. However, do not be alarmed if you took a tablet or two before you knew you were pregnant, since it has not been specifically shown to cause any harm either.

Do not take any over-the-counter analgesics more frequently than once every four hours. Never exceed the stated dose. Consult your doctor if it is necessary to continue taking painkillers for more than three days, if symptoms persist or if they recur frequently.

**What's Available?**   Actron, Alka-Seltzer and Andrews Resolve (especially for headache with upset stomach), Anadin, Anadin Extra, Anadin Maximum Strength, Anadin Paracetamol, APS Aspirin Tablets, Aspro, Aspro Clear, Aspro Clear Extra, Bayer Aspirin, Calpol Infant Suspension,

Calpol Six Plus, Calpol Under Six, Coda-Med, Codanin, Codis 500, Cupanol Over Six, Cuprofen Ibuprofen Tablets, Dentogen Ibuprofen Tablets, Disprin, Disprin Extra, Disprol, Junior Disprol Suspension, Fenning's Adult Powders, Fenning's Children's Cooling Powders, Hedex, Hedex Extra, Inoven, Junior Paraclear, Medised, Mrs Cullen's Powders, Nurofen, Panadeine, Panadol, Panadol Baby/ Infant Elixir, Panadol Extra, Panadol Junior, Paracelar, Paracetamol, Paracodol Propain, Proflex, Powerin, Solmin, Solpadeine, Syndol, Tramil 500, Veganin

**My Favourites**    Nurofen, Paracetamol soluble aspirin (both available from most chemists under 'own brand' labels), Solpadeine

## PERENNIAL RHINITIS

Having a cold once or twice a year, as most of us do, is bad enough – imagine what it would be like to have cold-like symptoms all the year round. Probably about one person in ten – children and adults – suffers in this way.

Rhinitis is simply an inflammation of the mucous membrane lining the nose and there are many possible causes. Seasonal rhinitis (see HAY FEVER p.66) occurs as an allergic reaction to pollens and other allergens around at a particular time of year – in between while the symptoms disappear.

In the case of perennial rhinitis, however, the nose remains inflamed and unpleasant symptoms – which may include a constantly blocked or runny nose, itchy eyes and frequent sneezing – persist. The sense of taste and smell can also be affected and the sufferer often feels generally 'under the weather'. If he or she experiences these symptoms for more than one hour in 24 on most days of the year, a diagnosis of perennial rhinitis can be made. Children who suffer from perennial rhinitis typically develop a 'nose crease' from constantly rubbing their itchy nose upwards, nose bleeds are quite common and dark circles under the eyes may be another sign.

So what causes these continuing symptoms? In a few

cases they will be due to a physical obstruction in the nose, such as polyps. Sometimes they will be a reaction to certain drugs, to changes in hormone levels – during pregnancy and at the menopause, for instance – or to changes in temperature and humidity. Irritating conditions at work, such as smoke or fumes, can also be responsible.

Most often, however, symptoms are due to an allergy – to animal fur and hair, for example, but especially to house-dust mites. These tiny creatures, invisible to the naked eye, exist in their millions in the furnishings, floors and bedding of even the cleanest home. They live on the dead skin cells that we shed constantly and each produces 40 faecal pellets a day – not a pretty thought! Fortunately, most of us co-exist quite happily with our house-dust mites, but these pellets are the trigger that provokes the allergic response and symptoms of perennial rhinitis in those susceptible.

Sufferers can minimise their problem by hoovering floors and furnishings and damp-dusting frequently, having the curtains and blankets cleaned regularly, covering mattresses with a plastic cover and using pillows and duvets made from artificial fibres rather than feathers. Polished boards or 'lino' are less of a mite trap than carpets. Mites thrive in warmth, so keep the bedroom cool and well aired. Smaller objects, such as children's fluffy toys, can be put into the deep freeze every so often – mites cannot survive at that temperature.

Many people who suffer from perennial rhinitis just put up with it – they think the symptoms are too trivial to bother their doctor with – or they try to treat themselves with medicines bought from the chemist, such as nasal decongestant sprays. Although these can be all right, used sparingly, for the short-term relief of the blocked nose at the end of a common cold, they are quite unsuitable for treating the long-term blocked nose of perennial rhinitis. Overuse of these sprays will soon damage the lining of the nose and actually make the condition worse with so-called 'rebound congestion'. Antihistamines bought over the counter will temporarily dry up a runny nose, but they will have no effect on a blocked nose and can cause drowsiness (for antihistamines to help ease rhinitis see 'What's Available?' under HAY FEVER p.66).

When nasal symptoms are persistent, it is important to consult a doctor, as there are several effective treatments that he or she can prescribe once the possible non-allergic causes already described have been excluded. Obviously, identifying the allergen so that the sufferer can avoid it as far as possible is helpful. Alternatively, anti-allergic, anti-inflammatory nasal sprays or drops, such as sodium cromoglycate or corticosteroids, if used consistently as directed, are very effective at both preventing and relieving symptoms. Sufferers often have, or have had, other allergic-type conditions, such as eczema or asthma, or these may run in the family. Successful treatment of rhinitis can also keep asthma attacks at bay.

So it is well worthwhile consulting your doctor if you seem to have a permanent head cold or 'hay fever' – these always have a limited duration. Perennial rhinitis does not, but modern treatments will relieve it.

**What's Available?**   Aller-Eze. See also HAY FEVER p.66

**Herbal Remedies**   Garlic (for the healing properties of garlic, see 'Herbal Remedies' under COLD, THE COMMON p.37), Herbelix Specific

# PERIOD PAIN
When young women get painful periods it's likely to be due to the womb going into a spasm. This causes a cramp-like pain as soon as the period starts, or a dull ache in the abdomen and back. Doctors call this primary dysmenorrhoea, to distinguish it from secondary dysmenhorroea, the kind of period pain that mainly affects older women.

Secondary dysmenorrhoea can be caused by disorders such as endometriosis (when the womb-lining tissue develops outside the womb), fibroids (benign tumours of the womb's muscular wall) or a continuing infection – pelvic inflammatory disease, for example.

In most cases painful periods are not a sign of ill health, but women who suddenly develop them should go to see their doctor, so that the cause can be treated appropriately. An ultrasound scan may occasionally be needed to detect – or rule out – any underlying disorder.

Sufferers from primary dysmenorrhoea sometimes have more of a chemical called prostaglandin in their menstrual flow than most women. The production of an egg, or ovum, in the middle of the month triggers the release of this excess prostaglandin, which sends pain signals to the brain – so when a woman doesn't ovulate she usually doesn't experience pain. That's why many women who suffer from painful periods are advised to take the contraceptive Pill, which generally works by preventing ovulation – this is a relatively straightforward form of bringing relief.

Painkillers also help you cope with period pain (see p.89 for product list). An anti-inflammatory one containing ibuprofen can inhibit the production of prostaglandin, which is why it can be so effective in relieving symptoms. Aspirin has the same effect. Mefenamic acid, which is an even more powerful prostaglandin dampener, has to be prescribed by your doctor. There are also antispasmodic medicines available on prescription – these will relieve symptoms by relaxing the uterine muscles. Some over-the-counter remedies contain antispasmodic agents – hyoscine hydrobromide, for example – as well as a mild anti-prostaglandin drug (paracetamol) and a mild diuretic (caffeine) to make you urinate more often. The diuretic helps relieve congestion in and around the womb.

Hot baths and hot water can also be soothing for period pain. Heat can help reduce muscle spasm, as can brisk exercise such as cycling, swimming and fast walking. A good, well-balanced diet with enough Vitamin B6 and other B vitamins is helpful, too (see VITAMINS p.213).

Once a woman has her first baby, the painful periods of the primary dysmenorrhoea kind will usually go for good.

**What's Available?**   Feminax, Librofem

# PILES

Piles, or haemorrhoids, are actually enlarged, worn-out veins – varicose veins that may feel rather like soft, spongy grapes. They're found in and around the lower rectum and anal canal at the very lowest end of the bowel, in a pad of tissue that is not unlike the lips found at the opposite end of the digestive system! Nature intended this soft tissue to be there because, when healthy, it makes a very good seal. But when the veins within it enlarge, becoming piles, a discharge of mucus from the anus can be just one of many distressing symptoms.

Doctors believe that at least half the people in Britain suffer from piles at some time in their life, although many are too embarrassed to seek advice. A susceptibility seems to run in families, perhaps due to an inherited weakness in the wall of the rectal blood vessels. The veins the walls contain, unlike veins elsewhere, do not have valves in them to aid the flow of blood. If anything increases the pressure on these rectal veins, they can become engorged and distended, just like varicose veins in the leg. So there is really no need to be embarrassed about having piles – the chances are that the doctor or pharmacist you consult will have had them too! They really are very common, even more so in men than in women. You are more likely to suffer from piles as you get older (especially if you are overweight), although quite young people can be troubled by them too.

There are many old wives' tales about the causes of piles. Despite popular belief, you do not get them by sitting on cold walls or hot radiators. Perhaps surprisingly, active sportsmen and women are prone to piles and, like varicose veins, they are a particular hazard of pregnancy. The weight of the developing baby can put pressure on the rectal veins, causing them to enlarge as the normal flow of blood is prevented. Fortunately, these piles usually subside after the baby's birth and treatment meanwhile can relieve the discomfort.

Some medicines, such as codeine and iron tablets, if taken regularly, can be constipating and so predispose to piles. However, chronic constipation, with the straining and increased pressure on the veins this brings, is one of the most common causes; as is a lack of fibre in the diet over many years.

If you have piles, the first sign you may notice is some bright red blood in the lavatory, or on the loo paper, after a bowel movement. It is always important to check with your doctor that this bleeding is caused by piles and not by some other condition.

'Internal' piles – also known as 'first degree' piles – which remain inside the anus are usually painless, but as the normal seal there is affected by the swollen veins, a constant, sometimes blood-stained, discharge may occur. There may also be itching and an uncomfortable aching feeling.

Second degree, 'external' piles, which prolapse through the anus, particularly when a motion is passed, tend to become inflamed, itchy and painful from time to time. They usually slip back, or can be gently pushed back, in between bowel movements. It may be easiest to do this while having a bath or using a bidet, when the area is lubricated with soap and your hands are clean.

If second degree piles are not treated, they may protrude permanently – when they are known as third degree piles – and cause considerable discomfort. Occasionally, a protruding pile will be gripped by the tight muscular band (sphincter) at the exit to the anus and become strangulated, which is very painful. If the blood inside the pile then clots, it will, in time, drop off – providing Nature's cure. Otherwise, rest in bed with the foot of the bed raised and an ice pack applied to the pile should relieve acute symptoms.

Less severe piles can often be cured completely by avoiding constipation and straining. So, if you have ever suffered from piles, or think you are likely to because they run in your family, do all you can to avoid becoming constipated. This means eating plenty of high-fibre foods – fresh fruit and vegetables, wholemeal bread and bran cereals, for instance. Fibre-containing tablets or drinks, such as Fybogel or Regulan, available from your chemist, can be helpful if you find it difficult to eat enough bran-type foods. Try also to cut down on salt and have plenty of watery or fruit drinks. This type of diet should keep your motions regular, well-formed and effortless. Laxatives are usually only advisable as a short-term measure.

If your symptoms persist, you can try some suppositories and/or ointments recommended by your pharmacist and follow their instructions. These mainly contain local anaesthetics such as lignocaine or cinchocaine to ease irritation, and astringents, bismuth subgallate for example, to help dry up piles and relieve inflammation. A suppository is usually inserted after each bowel movement and at night and in the morning. Suppositories should never be taken orally. Some are said to be safe to use in pregnancy, but always check this with your pharmacist. Your doctor may prescribe a short course of suppositories containing cortisone to relieve the inflammation and irritation, with perhaps an anaesthetic cream to ease the soreness. Again, sleeping with the foot end of the bed raised can also help.

If your piles keep recurring and being troublesome, your doctor will probably refer you to a surgeon for further advice. Injection treatment may be recommended for bleeding internal or less severe external piles. This involves injecting a special fluid into the dilated veins which causes them to shrink. You will be treated as an outpatient and, although the procedure may sound unpleasant, it is not painful and is usually very successful. In fact, it's one of the easiest and quickest forms of treatment.

As an alternative, cryosurgery – 'freezing' the veins – may be used, or constricting bands may be placed around the base of the veins. An operation under general anaesthetic, called 'Lord's procedure', can be very effective even for quite advanced piles. It involves a powerful stretching of the tight sphincter muscles around the anus. For severe third degree piles, however, many surgeons will advise removing them completely. This operation may cause discomfort for some time afterwards, but it should then solve the problem once and for all.

**What's Available?**   Anodesyn, Anusol, Hemocane Suppositories,   Nupercainol,   Lasonil,   Preparation   H Suppositories

**My Favourites**   Anusol, Preparation H

**Herbal Remedies**   Heemex, Nelsons Haemorrhoid Cream, Pileabs

## PRICKLY HEAT
Prickly heat is an extremely irritating skin rash which develops in hot weather. It occurs – more in some people than in others – when the small blood vessels under the skin widen as the temperature rises. The extra blood they then supply to the surface of the body acts as the body's radiator, allowing heat to escape, and the extra blood supplies the extra liquid which the sweat glands release as sweat. As the tissues swell with extra blood and tissue fluids, the skin becomes congested and the pores are squeezed and then blocked. The sweat builds up under the skin and causes a rash known as prickly heat or *Miliaria rubra*.

Sufferers from prickly heat will quickly recognise the emergence of small red pimples or blisters. The tissues look red because the small blood vessels are open wide, while the engorged tissues cause discomfort and feel prickly.

There's no simple, quick remedy, but if you can immerse yourself in water to keep cool, you should feel better. Covering yourself with light, white clothing will help and, obviously, keeping out of direct sunlight is a good idea, too. Calamine cream or lotions will cool the skin and antihistamine tablets can bring great relief.

**What's Available?**   Caladryl, Eurax Cream, Mycil Powder. See also HAY FEVER p.66 for antihistamines

**My Favourite**   Caladryl

## PSIORASIS
See DRY SKIN CONDITIONS p.59

## RHEUMATIC PAIN
Rheumatism is a general term describing pain which affects the muscles and joints. It covers many conditions, including osteoarthritis, a joint disorder, usually of late middle age, triggered by wear and tear in the joints included in which the protective, shock-absorbing, rubbery substance called cartilage between the bones wears away. Osteoarthritis is thought to affect almost 90% of people over the age of 60, mainly in the hips, knees and shoulders.

Fibrositis – inflammation of white fibrous tissue, especially that of muscle sheaths – also comes under the heading rheumatism. So does rheumatoid arthritis, caused by a progressive swelling of the joints and one of the most crippling of all the rheumatic diseases.

The most widely used pain-relieving treatment is aspirin, but other anti-inflammatory painkillers, ibuprofen, for example, can help (see PAINKILLERS p.89 for list of products containing these ingredients). Rheumatic pain can also be relieved with heat from a hot water bottle, rheumatic liniments and sprays: these treatments work by a process known as counter-irritation, something that causes superficial irritation of the skin and thereby relieves deep-seated pain. For more severe symptoms, your doctor can prescribe anti-inflammatory drugs or stronger painkillers, and perhaps arrange for physiotherapy. In extreme cases, an operation may be necessary to replace the damaged joint with an artificial one.

**What's Available?**   Algipan Rub and Spray, Bengue's Balsam, the Deep Heat range of products, especially Deep Heat Intensive Therapy and Deep Heat Deep Freeze Cold Gel, Lasonil, Massage Balm, Menthol and Wintergreen Rub, Proflex, PR Freeze Spray, PR Heat Spray, Radian-B Range, Hom Copper Ointment

**My Favourite**   The Deep Heat range

**Herbal Remedies**   Dr Valnet's Flexarome, Gonne Balm, Natural Olbas Oil, Nelsons Rhus Tox Cream

# SHINGLES

Shingles is a rash of blisters on the skin accompanied by a severe stinging pain, caused by a virus – the *Varicella zoster* virus – which is also responsible for chicken pox. Anyone who develops shingles will have had chicken pox in the past, sometimes without realising it, as one can have what is known as a 'subclinical' attack, in which no spots appear.

Antibodies to the virus develop in the bloodstream at the first infection and prevent further attacks of chicken pox. However, the virus is able to settle and lie dormant in a non-infectious state, in the 'junction boxes' of nerves supplying a part of the skin or – less commonly – muscles. Often it will cause no further trouble, but if it does, the result will be shingles.

All manner of events can trigger an attack. If you're emotionally or physically exhausted, or suffering from illness or injury – indeed, if your body's defences are not at their best for whatever reason, the virus can become active. The older you get, the more likely you are to develop shingles – of those who reach their eighties at least one in two will have suffered.

The first symptom is usually pain over the area of skin supplied by the nerves harbouring the virus. The most common place is around the side of the body, along a line following a rib. It can occur on both sides of the chest, but it is an old wives' tale that if it meets in the middle the outcome is fatal – that just isn't true.

To have the best chance of success any treatment should be given early on, preferably at the painful stage which can be when, or just before, the blisters appear.

Your doctor will sometimes prescribe a course of tablets which may help to lessen and shorten the attack. Antiviral applications to the affected area of skin can help and anaesthetic ointments or over-the-counter ointments containing calamine can also be soothing.

The surrounding skin should be kept clean to prevent other germs infecting the blisters, as this could interfere with healing and lead to scarring. Antibiotics may be needed if infection does occur.

**What's Available?**    Caladryl


# SINUS PAIN, NASAL CONGESTION AND CATARRH

Nasal congestion and catarrh – nasal discharge, or phlegm in the throat – are usually present for a few days during and after many infections of the nose and sinuses, especially the common cold (see p.33). The combination is a harmless but annoying problem that can be stubborn to shift and can also result in deafness if it builds up in the eustachian tubes (the tubes on either side at the back of the nose and throat, which lead to the ears).

One of the best ways of treating it is steam inhalation to help drainage. You can either do this by breathing the vapour being given off by plain hot – not boiling – water, or you can add decongestant capsules containing natural essential oils, such as pine or eucalyptus. Essential oils have a strong, pleasant odour and are extremely volatile. When exposed to air, they therefore give off a powerful vapour. Inhaling this helps give relief from catarrh, nasal congestion and sinus trouble and can loosen mucus. Do not let the vapour come into contact with the eyes.

You can also sprinkle the oils on to a handkerchief or tissue and breathe in the vapours that way. For older children and adults you can dab the oils on to bedding nearby, but avoiding the possibility of direct skin contact. Or for infants, a few drops in a jug of warm water placed in the room out of the child's reach, may give relief.

Tablets are also available over the counter to relieve sinus congestion and pain. These contain paracetamol and a drug called phenylpropanolamine hydrochloride which constricts blood vessels and thus helps ease congestion. Decongestant tablets and syrups can also be bought for blocked sinuses, stuffed-up nose and catarrh as part of cold and flu symptoms. These contain a decongestant such as pseudoephedrine hydrochloride.

You can also try sprays containing decongestants like oxymetazoline hydrochloride, which is used as a vasoconstrictor – a drug that causes narrowing of the walls of blood vessels to relieve congestion. But it's usually inadvisable to use nose drops for longer than ten days, as they can cause a 'rebound' swelling and damage to the nasal passages, making matters worse.

To insert nose drops, lie on your back on a bed with your head hanging over the edge and stay in that position for at least three minutes after inserting the drops. This prevents them simply running down the back of the nose into the throat and allows them to reach their destination – the sinuses.

If your symptoms become more severe and the sinuses are actually infected, the condition is then called sinusitis. Anyone who has ever suffered from this will remember all too well the typical throbbing headache which is made worse by bending over or blowing the nose. It's estimated that one in 200 colds leads to sinusitis.

The bones of the cheeks, forehead and back of the nose contain a hidden network of small caverns and channels – the sinuses – which help to make the bones lighter and give resonance to our voice. The mucus-secreting membrane that lines the nose continues on to form an interconnecting lining for all the sinuses and there are tiny holes in it which normally allow for free drainage and circulation of air. When germs or particles of dirt are inhaled, they lodge in the mucus; minute, moving 'hairs' called cilia then waft them to the back of the nose where they evaporate, are harmlessly swallowed or are blown out on to a handkerchief.

However, if the lining membrane of the sinuses becomes inflamed – which is quite common after a heavy cold – more mucus than usual is produced, the cilia cease to function properly, infected secretions build up, the tiny drainage holes may become blocked and acute sinusitis results. The pain can be similar to that caused by toothache and the affected sinus – along the cheekbone below the eye, or just above the eyebrow, for example – may be tender to the touch. The sufferer will probably feel generally unwell and have a nasty headache and a blocked nose. He or she may also have a temperature and greeny discharge from the nose or running down the back of the throat.

An allergy – to irritant fumes or smoking, for instance – can also cause the lining membrane of the sinuses to swell and lead to a recurrent form of sinusitis. Diving and underwater swimming may have the same effect, if water is forced up into the sinuses.

An acute attack of sinusitis can usually be successfully treated by rest, painkillers and steam inhalations three times a day to relieve the congestion and help the sinuses to drain. A constant and comfortable room temperature and a humid atmosphere (keep bowls of water by the radiators) should help, too.

Some people also swear by an age-old remedy for catarrh and sinus trouble – garlic, in the form of garlic oil capsules, available from most chemists and health food shops (see 'What's Available?' under COLD, THE COMMON, p.37, for suitable products).

Over-the-counter decongestant medicines may help treat sinusitis, but are not generally very effective and some can make you drowsy. Nose drops, if prescribed by a doctor, can be helpful. For a severe attack of sinusitis, your doctor may also prescribe antibiotics and, if symptoms do not improve or attacks recur, referral to a specialist may be necessary. Treatment may then include washing out the infected sinus under a local or general anaesthetic and finally an operation to improve the drainage system from the sinuses.

**What's Available?**   Actifed Syrup, Actifed Tablets, Afrazine Nose Drops, Aller-Eze Plus, Bengue's Balsam, Catarrh-Ex, Catarrh Pastilles, Congesteze, Cupal Baby Chest Rub, Dimotapp Elixir, Dimotapp Elixir Paediatric, Dimotapp LA, Dristan Decongestant Tablets, Dristan Spray, Famel Catarrh and Throat Pastilles, Fenox Nasal Drops, Flurex, Karvol Decongestant Capsules, Mentholatum Vapour Rub, Mucron, Mucron Junior Syrup, Otrivine, Penetrol Catarrh Lozenges, Penetrol Inhalant, Sinex Decongestant Nasal Spray, Sinutab, Sudafed Elixir, Sudafed Tablets, Throaties Catarrh Pastilles, Triogesic, Triominic

**My Favourites**   Sudafed Tablets, Sinex Decongestant Nasal Spray

**Homoeopathic Remedies**   Silicea, and for Catarrh, Arsen. Alb., Kali. Bich., Pulsatilla.

**Herbal Remedies**   Garlic, Dr Valnet's Climarone Inhalant, Herbelix Specific, Natural Olbas Oil Inhalant Decongestant, Olbas Pastilles

## SLEEPLESSNESS
Sleep has been the subject of a great deal of research and the results, for insomniacs, are reassuring. It seems that, in the long run, Nature ensures that we get the sleep we need and there is no hard and fast rule on how much we should have – individuals differ considerably in this. What matters most is how you feel the next day – if you are alert and efficient, although you have had only five hours sleep, then that was enough for you and comparisons with friends can cause

unnecessary worry. Remember, too, that the need for sleep lessens as we grow older.

It is also reassuring to know that even a prolonged period of unsatisfactory sleep will do no serious harm, although you may feel a bit tired and irritable and be less efficient than usual. Eventually the body will catch up on its sleep debt.

Experiments have shown that poor sleepers in fact often sleep more than they think they do, although perhaps not as deeply as others. During sleep, children grow and the body's worn-out tissues are renewed. Sleep is needed to relieve mental fatigue more than physical fatigue – just resting in bed will do this.

It is not yet known whether the sleep induced by sleeping pills is as restorative as natural sleep. Sleeping pills can be useful when taken for a short time, to re-establish a pattern of sleep after a crisis, say, or to relieve anxiety about not sleeping. But dependency can easily develop and can be difficult to break. A 'rebound' insomnia is also common after stopping the pills, making it very tempting to take them again.

Elderly people will often ask their doctor for sleeping pills just because they find lying awake boring and feel they should be asleep – not because they are suffering any ill effects. However, fitful sleep is usual as we grow older and sleeping pills may cause confusion and make falls more likely.

Nearly everyone has times when they sleep badly – a hectic day at work, a difficult time with the children, problems of all kinds leave us feeling worked up or on edge, and make it hard to relax. But for a few, sleep is a lasting problem. They may find it difficult to fall asleep, or they may wake up frequently or very early. Twice as many women suffer as men, especially those with an anxious personality.

Depression is a common cause of sleeplessness and, if severe, both can be relieved by antidepressants. Pain – from arthritis for example – can interfere with sleep (try pain-relievers before bed, not sleeping pills – see PAINKILLERS p.89 for product list); so too can breathing difficulties and some medicines. Alcohol, tea, coffee and cigarettes are all stimulants, so should be avoided before going to bed, whereas a light snack or a milky drink can help induce sleep. A warm bath before going to bed can be very relaxing. And a good read in bed will eventually lead to drowsiness.

As other aids to better sleep, establish a regular routine of meal times, of getting up early and of going to bed at about the same time every night – this helps the body's 'internal clock'. Make sure your bed is comfortable and the room warm, but not too warm. Imagine a peaceful scene and concentrate on relaxing each part of your body in turn. A special relaxation or sleep cassette can help you learn this technique. Some daily exercise in the fresh air will make sound sleep more likely and talking over any problems with a sympathetic person can relieve one cause of insomnia – worry.

If night sweats during the menopause disturb your sleep, hormone replacement therapy can help. If noise is a problem, try ear plugs. Overweight people tend to sleep better and losing weight can mean losing sleep – but obviously it's best to get the balance right here!

There are herbal remedies available for sleeplessness and these may be worth a try. Above all, remember that fear of not sleeping in itself can prevent sleep, so try not to let lying awake worry you – just sit up and read the most boring book you can find and you should soon fall asleep!

**Homoeopathic Remedies**   Noctura, Avena Sativa comp.

**Herbal Remedies**   Kalms Tablets, Natracalm, Naturest

## SORE THROAT

Sore throat remedies grab a multi-million pound share of the over-the-counter medicine market – a £71 million share, in fact! Yet there's little evidence that they reduce inflammation or shorten the duration of the infection. Nevertheless many people find the lozenges and gargles soothing and seem to be more than willing to pay for them. The medicines contain a variety of substances, including antiseptics such as domiphen bromide, local anaesthetics such as lignocaine hydrochloride, or antibacterial agents such as tyrothricin. Don't give throat lozenges to children under three, who may choke if the sweet sticks in their throat.

A sore throat is an infection making the throat red and sore, most often due to a viral infection which clears up by itself after three or four days. Pain can be relieved by taking soluble aspirin or your preferred painkiller (see PAINKILLERS p.89 for product list). Avoid smoking if your throat is very sore.

The exact cause of a sore throat can only be established as other symptoms develop. And there are many possible causes – it may be due to a virus and be the start of a cold or flu. It is also one of the first signs of German measles, pharyngitis or tonsillitis – the latter two of which may need antibiotics. So if sore throat symptoms persist, consult your doctor.

**What's Available?**   Antiseptic Throat Pastilles, Bradosol Lozenges, Bradosol Plus, Coldrex Hot Blackcurrant and Lemon Drinks, Dequacaine, Dequadin, Famel Catarrh and Throat Pastilles, Famel Honey and Lemon Cough Pastilles, Meggozones, Merocaine, Merocets, Merothol, Oraldene, Throaties, Tixylix, Tyrocane, Tyrocane Junior Antiseptic Lozenges, Tyrozets, Ulc-Aid Lozenges, Valda Pastilles, Vicks Chloraseptic Sore Throat Lozenges, Vicks Chloraseptic Sore Throat Spray, Zensyls

**My Favourite**   Merocets

**Homoeopathic Remedies**   Aconite, Arsen. Alb., Bryonia

**Herbal Remedies**   Olbas Pastilles

# STICKY EYES

Many of us will know what it's like to wake up in the morning with itchy, 'gritty'-feeling eyes and perhaps the eyelids stuck together. Underneath, the eyelids will be red and inflamed and the whites of the eyes probably bloodshot. Blinking may be painful and bright light distressing.

Conjunctivitis, as this condition is called, is very common and children are particularly prone to it. The symptoms are due to an inflammation of the conjunctiva – the delicate membrane that covers the whites of the eyes and the inner surfaces of the upper and lower eyelids. Where the membrane turns back on itself to cover both surfaces of the lids, sacs are formed, and small particles may collect here and irritate the conjunctiva – one cause of conjunctivitis.

Another possible cause is a viral or bacterial infection. Alternatively, the inflammation may be brought on by an allergic reaction – to pollens, animal hairs, cosmetics or the cleansing lotions used for contact lenses, for example.

It's perhaps surprising that conjunctivitis is not even more common than it is, since the eye is constantly exposed to various irritants and germs. Fortunately, the conjunctival sac is not an ideal breeding ground for germs, partly because of the cleansing effect of tear fluid. If a tear duct is blocked, then inflammation commonly develops and the duct will probably have to be unblocked.

If, as well as being red and sore, the eyes are gummed up with sticky discharge – including perhaps some yellow pus – this usually means that the conjunctivitis is due to a virus or bacteria. The discharge will be particularly noticeable first thing in the morning, having accumulated during the night. The sufferer may also have a cold or other infection such as, in the case of a child, measles. The discharge from the eyes is contagious, so keep handkerchiefs, towels, flannels and pillow cases separate to avoid spreading the germs to others. Your doctor will probably prescribe antibiotic eye drops and/ or ointment to apply several times a day – be sure to wash your hands both before and after doing so. The condition should improve within about four days – if not, referral to an eye specialist may be advised.

Another condition which causes irritating, sticky eyes is blepharitis, which I discussed earlier when talking about dandruff (see p.53).

Conjunctivitis due to an allergy such as hay fever will usually produce a watery discharge and can often be relieved by special preventive eye drops such as Opticrom, available on prescription, or other soothing eye lotions containing cooling witch-hazel and small amounts of anti-septics. Dark glasses can also help.

Sometimes town-dwellers will suffer from a persistent type of mild though distressing conjunctivitis – known as 'urban eye' – caused by irritant fumes and dust. Bathing the eyes twice a day with a solution of one teaspoonful of bicarbonate of soda dissolved in one pint of recently boiled and cooled water can relieve the symptoms. Use a separate piece of cotton wool for each eye, bathing the edges of the closed lids, working inwards towards the nose.

It's best to avoid eye make-up during any attack of conjunctivitis – in fact it's possible that make-up is the cause. Likewise, if you wear contact lenses, revert to your spectacles while your eyes are inflamed and ask your doctor's or ophthalmic optician's advice on future use. And if your eyes become painful or your vision is affected, always consult your doctor without delay. These symptoms could indicate that there was inflammation within the eye and in that case urgent examination and treatment, probably by a specialist, would be required without delay.

**What's Available?**    Optrex Eye Lotion, Optrex Clearine Eye Drops (for minor eye irritations)


# SUNBURN
While a small amount of sunshine on the skin is beneficial – it supplies Vitamin D and helps to keep the more harmful germs that live on the skin at bay – there is no longer any

doubt that continuous and prolonged exposure to the sun or the rays of a sunbed can be harmful.

This harm is observed in all sorts of ways – the skin ages prematurely, with wrinkling and dark brown blemishes, often accompanied by an ugly thickening of patches of the top skin layers, called solar keratosis. Skin changes that we notice as we get older, wrinkles and loss of elasticity, are now believed to be mainly due to damage from the sun. About 70% of this skin damage, which may take years to show, probably occurs in childhood, as a young child's skin is thinner than that of an adult and more likely to burn.

Each time the skin is burnt, the damage accumulates and the risk of skin cancer developing in the future increases. Over-exposure to the ultra-violet rays of the sun makes the skin red, hot and sore. Higher doses lead to inflammation and swelling; even greater exposure leads to burning, blistering and peeling as the epidermis – the outer layer of skin – disintegrates. Very bad sunburn damages the skin so much that it cannot carry out its usual functions. The heat absorbed from over-exposure to the sun can stop the body's temperature gauge from working properly, resulting in sunstroke, which has been known to kill.

Yet nobody really need suffer from sunburn. Prevention is always better than cure. It's worth remembering that you can get burnt even on cloudy days – 80% of ultra-violet rays get through cloud and water. Always try to use a protective cream. Proprietary suntan products, such as the Uvistat range or the Sun E45 range, which protects against UVA/UVB rays, are labelled with SPFs – sun protection factors – devised to tell you how much protection you can expect. They work by absorbing, reflecting or scattering the sun's rays – the higher the number, the more protection the product should give.

Remember, too, that babies and young children are particularly vulnerable to the sun's harmful rays, so always use a sun protection cream designed for their delicate skins. Babies under six months old should be kept out of the sun anyway, not just because of the risk of sunburn, but because heatstroke can be even more dangerous.

Sticking to the rule of avoiding the sun between 11 a.m. and 4 p.m. – when ultra-violet radiation is at its most intense because the sun is directly overhead – may not necessarily be the best safeguard: times vary according to geography and seasonal changes. So a good tip is to watch your shadow. When it's the same height as you are, the sun's rays are at an angle of 45° and therefore less dangerous – provided, of course, that you use an adequate sunscreen. If your shadow is shorter, you're more likely to burn.

If you do suffer from sunburn, the painful effects don't normally last for more than a few days, followed by itching as the skin heals. Lotions containing calamine or aloe vera with perhaps menthol, phenol or camphor have a cooling effect on the skin. Blisters should not be burst and you should drink plenty of water just in case you have become dehydrated. If the skin is burnt or peeling, stay out of the sun until it has healed completely. If symptoms are severe, always consult a doctor.

**What's Available?**   Acriflex, Cal-A-Cool, Caladryl, Lacto Calamine, Lana-Sting Spray, Medicaid, RBC, Solarcaine, Sudocrem, Sun E45 range, Uvistat range, Witch Doctor

**My Favourite**   Caladryl

**Homoeopathic Remedies**   Combudoron Lotion

# TEETHING

Babies cut their first teeth, on average, at about the age of six months and don't complete their set of 20 baby or milk teeth until they're around two to three years old. The first don't usually give any trouble, but when the back teeth come through, they can cause pain. Some babies sail through teething without a murmur, while others aren't quite so fortunate.

Teething trouble is pretty easy to spot – if your baby is

grizzly or upset, dribbling more than usual, has a red cheek or is gnawing everything in reach, then it's likely that teething is the cause. But if you have any doubts at all, it's best to get medical advice so as not to blame teething and overlook any real illness.

Special teething gels are available to relieve the baby's discomfort. These usually contain antiseptics such as cetyl-pyridinium chloride to prevent infection, as well as a local anaesthetic like lignocaine hydrochloride to numb any pain. Teething gel can be applied using a small pad of cotton wool or a clean finger and then rubbed gently on to the baby's gums. Repeat after 20 minutes if necessary. If your child is in great discomfort you can also use paracetamol infant suspensions to relieve the pain.

While we're talking about teeth, you may not realise that you can help look after your baby's teeth even before they appear. Don't allow sweet substances to stay in contact with his or her gums for long periods. This means not using baby drinks in bottles as a comforter and not dipping dummies in sweet syrups or honey.

**What's Available?**   Anbesol, Calgel, Calpol Infant Suspension, Cupanol Under Six, Dentinox Teething Gel, Fenning's Children's Cooling Powders, Junior Paraclear, Teejel Gel (use only under professional guidance if the child is sensitive to or is currently being prescribed aspirin)

**My Favourite**   Calpol Infant Suspension

**Homoeopathic Remedies**   Chamomilla Granules, Chamomilla 3 × Drops or Pilules, Nelsons Teething Granules

# TOOTHACHE
No matter how often we visit the dentist, our teeth are constantly under threat from our diet. We tend to eat more sugar than is good for us, and after every meal, snack or drink containing carbohydrates, food sugars in our mouth

are converted by plaque bacteria into acids which attack tooth enamel (its protective layer) for 40 minutes or longer. This can lead to decay spreading down a tooth's root canal to the nerve, causing inflammation and pain.

As well as decay, toothache can be caused by such things as a cracked filling or fractured tooth, even an abscess, so any type of pain in a tooth or in the gums should always be checked out by a dentist. Aspirin (not for children), paracetamol and ibuprofen can all be effective in treating dental pain if you have to wait for an appointment (see PAINKILLERS p.89 for list of products containing these ingredients). Oil of cloves applied to the aching tooth by means of a soaked piece of cotton wool can help numb the pain, too.

To help prevent further attacks of toothache, brush your teeth regularly. The use of dental floss is recommended, as I mentioned when talking about gum disease (see p.63), and you can also try a dental health gum after eating and drinking. This helps neutralise the teeth-attacking acids and so can help prevent tooth decay. Many millions of people throughout the world now drink artificially fluoridated water and millions more live in areas where the water contains natural fluoride. The addition of fluoride to water supplies is a frequent cause of confusion and controversy. Many people do not realise that some fluoride is naturally present in almost all water supplies and in most foods, so we ingest a certain amount each day. Usually, though, it is not enough to give our teeth as much protection as they need. Fluoridation of the water does not therefore involve adding a 'foreign' substance – it is simply a controlled means of adjusting the amount of fluoride to the most beneficial level. Experts now agree that although, as with most things, too much fluoride can be harmful, the recommended amount of one part per million (1 ppm) in the drinking water has no harmful effects.

Fluoride is an active ingredient in many toothpastes and you can buy fluoride drops and tablets over the counter to help protect children's teeth. So those who are against the addition of fluoride to the water supply ask why we cannot just use these products? The answer is that in order to be most effective, fluoride must be available continuously – during pregnancy for the mother-to-be and, for almost everyone, from birth through to late adolescence, so that it becomes built into the structure of the teeth as they develop and grow. However well-intentioned they may be, few parents could maintain the necessary continuity – giving each of their children a daily dose of fluoride for say 18 years, quite apart from the expense. Fluoride toothpaste, although helpful, only acts on the surface of the tooth, so is not as effective at preventing decay, though very good, nevertheless.

At present about 7,000 sets of dentures are supplied to school-age children in this country each year and one in three adults has no natural teeth left. In the few areas in Britain where the water has been fluoridated for many years – Birmingham is one example – tooth decay amongst children has been reduced by 50% and the number of extractions needed has dropped dramatically. The middle-aged who have lived in fluoridated areas since childhood also have much less decay, so the benefits are lasting.

Although avoiding sugary foods and in-between meal snacks will do much to prevent decay, our teeth are still constantly under attack from acid-producing germs. Teeth with fluoride built into their substance are undoubtedly better equipped for the fight. The earlier additional fluoride can be given, the better – preferably from soon after birth in the form of drops. Fluoride tablets can be taken when a child is older and should, ideally, be continued all the time that milk teeth and permanent teeth are growing. Dosage of drops and tablets will depend on the child's age and how much fluoride is present in the local drinking water, so consult your dentist or pharmacist first.

**What's Available?**   Dentogen Clove Oil Liquid, Dentogen Ibuprofen Tablets, Endekay Dental Health Gum, Endekay Fluoride Tablets and Drops, Oil of Cloves

**My Favourites**   For toothache: 'Own brand' Oil of Cloves.
For adding fluoride: Endekay Tablets and Drops

## TRAVEL SICKNESS

Travel sickness can be a misery not only for sufferers but
for those travelling with them. It can easily ruin what
started out as a pleasant journey or family outing. Travel
sickness can last up to 72 hours on a very long journey, but
it can also stop very quickly once the journey has finished.

Symptoms such as nausea and vomiting, loss of appetite,
sweating, feeling faint and looking pale, even greenish,
during a car, sea or air journey are actually brought on by
the disturbance to the balance mechanism of the inner ear
caused by motion. The movement of the vehicle upsets the
link between what the eyes see and what the balance
mechanism of the inner ear feels – hence the alternative
name of 'motion sickness'. The eyes adjusts to the changes
in the movement, whereas the inner ear doesn't, so the
signals from the eyes and the ears don't quite add up.

Medicines for combating travel sickness are known as
anti-emetics. They are drugs such as meclozine hydrochloride, an antihistamine, and they reduce the sensitivity of the
vomiting centre in the brain. Some of the anti-travel
sickness medicines cause drowsiness, so always read
instructions carefully. Some aren't recommended during
pregnancy, either, so do check with your pharmacist or
doctor if you're pregnant and suffer from travel sickness.
For most benefit, travel sickness medicines should be taken
at least one hour before your journey starts.

You can reduce the risk of travel sickness by following
some self-help measures. Don't have a large meal or
alcoholic drink before a journey, don't allow smoking in the
car and keep windows open if possible.

Children's ears tend to be sensitive, making them more
prone to travel sickness than adults, so if you have children
who suffer, don't talk about being sick in front of them, and
provide plenty of distractions – games, toys, puzzles, etc. If

possible, travel at night when they're more likely to fall asleep – and if all else fails do take some waterproof bags with you!

**What's Available?**    Kwells, Sea-Legs, Stugeron, Q-Mazine Syrup

**My Favourite**    Stugeron

**Homoeopathic Remedies**    Nelsons Travel Sickness Tablets


# URTICARIA
More often known as hives or nettle rash, urticaria is a very common skin condition which affects one in five people at some time in their lives. Women are particularly prone, perhaps because of hormonal influences. With 'ordinary' urticaria, weals – intensely itchy raised marks on the surface of the skin – suddenly develop. They are usually short-lived, lasting for a few hours or days, but may last longer. The weals can be any size, appear anywhere on the sufferer's body and may be numerous. They are usually pale in the middle and red around the edges and are due to dilation of the capillaries – small blood vessels under the skin – which makes their walls more permeable and enables clear fluid called serum to leak out. If enough serum leaks out, blisters may form.

If deeper tissues are involved, a more severe type of urticaria known as angio-oedema may occur. Then the swellings are much larger, commonly affecting the face, eyelids, hands, forearms and throat and sometimes causing serious breathing difficulties. Joints in the arms and legs may also become inflamed and painful. About half the people who suffer from ordinary urticaria have recurrent attacks of angio-oedema too.

So what causes this reaction in the blood vessels? Often it is due to an increased circulation of histamine – a chemical normally present in the body. This increase can be triggered by many factors, including various foods, drugs and inhalants such as pollens, house dust and animal 'dander' – skin flakes which the animal sheds naturally and various chemicals which its body gives off. Two foods that are frequently responsible are shellfish and strawberries – so urticaria is a hazard of summer for those susceptible. Other foods that may produce the reaction include eggs, nuts, chocolate, tomatoes, pork, milk and yeast. Artificial colourings and preservatives can do so, too.

Aspirin can also be a cause of urticaria, or it can aggravate it. Penicillin is another possible culprit, as are the non-steroidal anti-inflammatory drugs often given to treat arthritis.

Sometimes contact with certain substances will bring the symptoms on – cosmetics are one example. Insect stings can also cause this type of reaction, which may even be life-threatening if the breathing is affected (see BITES AND STINGS p.25).

People whose urticaria occurs in response to triggers such as these are often but not always allergy-prone individuals – sufferers from hay fever, asthma or eczema for example – and the tendency can run in families. Anxiety may also play a part.

Other constituents in the body – called catechol amines – can, by irritating the tissues surrounding them, have the same effect on the blood vessels as histamine and almost anything can act as the trigger in this allergic-type of urticaria. I had it once after eating raw fish in a foreign restaurant, for example, but it may also have been due to the monosodium glutamate used as a taste-enhancer.

It can therefore be exceedingly difficult to track down – in order to avoid – the cause if the attacks are recurrent. In fact three out of four people are unable to do so, in spite of persistent detective work.

Some more unusual forms of urticaria have a physical cause. Cold winds or rain, or just immersing the hands or bathing in cold water, can cause weals to appear in susceptible people. If an ice cube on the skin produces a weal, this confirms the diagnosis of 'cold urticaria' – the type that's induced by the cold.

Some people develop weals when exposed to sunlight – 'solar urticaria'. Others may suffer from 'pressure urticaria' – deep, painful, non-itchy swellings which occur about two hours after some particular pressure on the skin. The hands may swell, for instance, after carrying a heavy shopping bag, or the balls of the feet after spending some time on a ladder.

Another strange form of urticaria is called dermographism, loosely 'translated' as skin writing. A mild, stroking pressure – with a fingernail for example – will produce a temporary, raised line with reddened edges. The skin can literally be used as a drawing board.

Fortunately, however, most cases of urticaria tend to resolve themselves in due course, and in the meantime antihistamine tablets prescribed by your doctor or recommended by your pharmacist usually relieve the symptoms and keep the condition under control. For mild cases, soothing creams containing antihistamine which stop the effects of histamine on the blood vessels beneath the skin, or creams and lotions containing calamine lotion help calm down any swelling and itching by cooling the skin, especially if these preparations contain menthol, phenol or camphor.

If angio-oedema is severe and breathing becomes difficult, emergency treatment by injection may be necessary to reduce the swelling.

Urticaria can occur as part of some other underlying condition – thyroid disease, for example. So if the cause is not immediately apparent, or you have more than one attack, or are concerned, do consult your doctor. He or she may wish to do blood tests and other investigations or refer you to a skin specialist.

**What's Available?**   Anethane Itch Soothing Cream, Caladryl, Cal-a-Cool, Eurax, Lanacane, Lana-Sting Spray and Creme, Q-Mazine Syrup, RBC, Triludan, Triludan Forte

**My Favourite**   Caladryl

**Homoeopathic Remedies** Apis. Mel., Combudoron Lotion, Lycopodium, Nat. Mur., Sulphur,

# VERRUCAS

Plantar warts on the feet, also known as verrucas, as opposed to common warts (see WARTS p.121), tend to grow inwards rather than outwards because of the constant pressure on them from standing and walking. Verrucas normally occur on the sole of the foot and are moist. The skin surface is rough and the shape irregular. They often have tiny black centres, appear in groups and become painful if they press on a nerve.

Verrucas are caused by a virus entering the foot, possibly via a slight area of damage – in the same way as common warts – and are very infectious, particularly among children. The virus loves warmth and moisture – and soggy feet! – so is easily passed on in such places as swimming pools and showers. If you have verrucas, therefore, you shouldn't go barefoot until they have cleared up. Many swimming pools now provide plastic socks for children with verrucas to wear so as to avoid infecting others.

Verrucas can be treated with over-the-counter remedies which usually contain a keratolytic – salicylic acid, for example – to soften the verruca so that it can be cut out or pulled off. If possible, cover the verruca with a ring-pad plaster to protect the surrounding skin. Put a small quantity of the ointment or paint on the verruca, then cover it with a plaster for two to three days. After several applications, the verruca should separate from the surrounding healthy tissue. If this doesn't happen within about two weeks, consult your doctor or chiropodist.

After a few days of treatment, the verruca will probably appear white or blanched. This is perfectly normal and indicates that the treatment is working well.

You can also get rid of verrucas with another form of treatment which doesn't require the use of sticking plasters. Buy a non-keratolytic paint such as Glutarol which contains glutaraldehyde, a disinfectant working directly on the wart virus, inhibiting its activity. It also exerts a powerful anhidrotic, or anti-sweating effect, which reduces the tendency of warts and verrucas to spread, so helping to minimise the risk of cross-infection.

Other methods of removing verrucas if they become painful are cryotherapy – 'freezing' them with liquid nitrogen; 'burning' with an electric cautery; or scraping them out with a scalpel called a curette. Often a local anaesthetic will be given first to numb the surrounding area. A chiropodist is usually the best person to consult about recurrent or persistent verrucas.

Sufferers from diabetes should always consult a doctor about foot problems because they can more easily pick up infection.

**What's Available?**   Compound W, Cupal Verruca Treatment, Duofilm, Glutarol, Salactol

**My Favourite**   Compound W

# WARTS
Much folklore is associated with warts, and some intriguing forms of treatment. One 'cure' was to rub your warts with stones. The stones then had to be wrapped up and left at the crossroads on the way to church. If another person picked up the stones, he would heal your warts by acquiring them himself!

Quite simply, warts are small, dry lumps of skin often seen on the hands, knees and face and they develop when a virus invades the skin cells and causes them to multiply very quickly. They're spread through contact with skin that's been shed from a wart or by the virus coming into contact with damaged skin, particularly if it is warm and moist. That's why it's advisable to use only your own towels until your warts have cleared, to reduce the risk of spreading the condition to other members of your household.

Warts are a nuisance as they can be so ugly, but they're normally harmless and, if untreated, most of these 'common warts' will eventually disappear of their own accord – although this may not happen for many years.

The virus's incubation period varies from a few weeks to several months, as it often lies dormant for some time. That's why warts can erupt months after the initial infection. For the same reason warts can reappear after treatment has apparently been successful. Adults will usually have developed some immunity to the virus over the years and are less likely to catch warts than children.

If you find common warts unsightly or annoying, you can apply a solution or cream every day to get rid of them. Most contain a caustic such as acetic acid, which destroys any tissue it's applied to, or a keratolytic drug such as salicylic acid to soften the wart and loosen it. Keeping the wart(s) covered with a plaster may speed up the treatment process, but remember, there's no immediate cure and treatment with one of these products can still take weeks to complete. Make sure, too, that you follow instructions very carefully, because these remedies can make the skin surrounding the wart very sore. Immediately wash off any solvent accidentally applied to surrounding skin to avoid painful acid burns.

If you have a wart that doesn't respond to an over-the-counter treatment, ask your doctor for advice. Other methods of removing warts are the same as those for verrucas (see p.120).

Women can develop genital warts in or around the vagina or on the cervix and men can have them on the penis. These warts are usually transmitted during sexual intercourse but may occur for other reasons.

Although genital warts are also due to a virus infection, a slightly different strain is probably responsible for each type of wart. Most genital warts develop from a root-like base below the surface of the skin and all have their own blood supply, so this must be taken into account when treating them. Never treat any warts on the genitals or around the anus with over-the-counter remedies.

Some wart-like brown or black eruptions not due to a virus are the so-called 'seborrhoeic' or senile warts which many people develop on their body, temple or scalp as they get older. These usually cause no problems, but they can sometimes itch severely. It's best to have them examined by a doctor who may advise removing them.

In general, it's advisable to let a doctor examine any wart when it first appears and especially, as with moles, if it changes in size or colour, or begins to bleed. But usually warts remain nothing but an annoying blemish.

For advice on plantar warts on the feet, also called verrucas, see VERRUCAS p.120.

**What's Available?**   Compound W, Cupal Wart Solvent, Duofilm, Glutarol, Salactol, Salatac Gel

**My Favourite**   Compound W

# WORMS
Threadworms (Enterobius) are like little strands of white cotton – hence the name. They are less than 1.5 cm long and can be seen wriggling in the faeces. Horrible as they sound, they are a very common problem, particularly in children. It is estimated that up to 40% of children below the age of ten are infected with threadworms, though many may not show the 'itching' symptoms generally associated with them.

Threadworms produce large numbers of tiny eggs that cannot be seen with the naked eye. The eggs are present in house dust, they stick to clothing, carpets, towels and bed linen and can also be picked up in garden soil or on unwashed vegetables and salads. They are spread by eating contaminated food or by hand contact. If another person should touch an infected person's hands when eggs are present and subsequently put his or her hands into the mouth, then he or she will also become infected as a result of swallowing the eggs. The eggs then hatch in the lower bowel and at night a female worm starts to lay her eggs just outside the anus. She can lay up to 10,000 eggs, which can cause severe itching.

The wriggling of threadworms irritates the anus and their presence slightly inflames it. This normally makes the sufferer scratch and so pick up eggs on the hands and under the fingernails. The most common sign of threadworms is scratching of the bottom, particularly at night and first thing in the morning. When the scratching takes place solely during the night, as sometimes happens, it may just cause a disturbance of sleep and hence daytime irritability – the itching itself may not be apparent. Some sufferers show no signs of infection, in which case it is a question of spotting the worms in the motions in order to detect their presence.

Threadworms are very common and appear even in the cleanest households, so there's no need to feel embarrassed about consulting your doctor. They only affect humans, never pets. And although they can be uncomfortable, they are generally harmless and do not usually cause any long-term damage.

You can buy a remedy from the chemist containing mebendazole, which kills threadworms, or piperazine, which is one of a number of substances that paralyse the worms so they can then be passed out in the faeces. These treatments are usually effective, but you should follow the instructions on the packet exactly. If the problem recurs, then everyone in your household should take a course of the medicine at the same time (your pharmacist will advise you on the correct dosage for each individual), as they may be harbouring worms themselves without necessarily having any symptoms. If this is the case, the worms can, in a variety of ways, be continually passed from person to person. So if, after treatment, your symptoms return, gather your courage and bring up the subject with everyone sharing your home – you may find they've been suffering silently, too.

Make sure that everyone scrubs their fingers and nails with a brush after each visit to the toilet and before each meal. Disinfect – by washing thoroughly – the toilet seat, toilet handle or chain and door handle regularly, as well as making sure you dust and vacuum bedrooms thoroughly.

Roundworms (ascariasis) can also be treated by piperazine. These worms are one of the largest parasites – they can be 10–30 cm long, look like earthworms and can block the intestine. They're transmitted by eggs found in contaminated raw food or in soil. Fortunately, they're rare. The sufferer may inexplicably lose weight or suffer other symptoms – a cough is not uncommon. When the doctor takes a blood test, the results should strongly suggest the diagnosis. Occasionally, an adult worm, not unlike an earthworm, may be passed in the faeces or even vomited up. But don't be alarmed – as I said, it's rare, thank goodness.

The roundworm is usually eradicated by a single dose of a medicine containing piperazine, whereas threadworms may need several days' treatment, as instructed, and phases of treatment may sometimes be separated by a week or more.

**What's Available?**   Expelix, Ovex TM, Pripsen

**My Favourite**   Pripsen

# A–Z of Over-the-Counter Medicines

To make it easy for you to find out about a medicine, I have listed them here with a short description and any relevant comments. The recommended dosages and other instructions are also given.

NOTE: where appropriate, dosages are given in millilitres (ml). One 5 ml spoonful = one teaspoonful; one 15 ml spoonful = one tablespoonful

## Acetoxyl 2.5 and 5

Greaseless, odourless, antiseptic medications containing benzoyl peroxide for the treatment of acne. It may be necessary to change to Acetoxyl 5 as the skin becomes accustomed to treatment with the milder Acetoxyl 2.5. Apply once daily after washing the affected area.                    STIEFEL

## Acnegel and Acnegel Forte

Acne gels containing benzoyl peroxide, invisible on the skin. Acnegel Forte has a higher percentage of benzoyl peroxide. Apply once a day after washing affected area.
                              STIEFEL

## Acriflex

Soothing cream with chlorhexidine – an antiseptic – for the treatment of minor burns and scalds, scratches, cuts and abrasions, sunburn blisters and cracked skin. For general use, apply freely and smooth gently into the skin. For cuts, abrasions, burns etc., spread freely and, if necessary, cover with a dressing.
                         EVANS MEDICAL

## Actal

Antacid tablets containing alexitol sodium for relief from indigestion, stomach upset, heartburn or dyspepsia due to over-acidity. For adults only:

allow two tablets to dissolve on the tongue as required.

STERLING HEALTH

## Actifed Compound Linctus

Linctus for the relief of dry cough and other symptoms that accompany coughs and colds, such as runny nose, catarrh, nasal congestion and blocked-up sinuses. Contains an antihistamine, triprolidine hydrochloride; a decongestant, pseudoephedrine hydro-chloride; and dextro-methorphan hydrobromide, a cough-suppressant. May cause drowsiness. As with all medicines, if you're pregnant or currently taking any other medicine, consult your doctor or pharmacist before taking this product.

Dosage, three times a day: Adults and children over 12 – two 5 ml spoonfuls. Children 6–12 years – one 5 ml spoonful; 2–5 years – half a 5 ml spoonful. WELLCOME

## Actifed Expectorant

An expectorant to help loosen stubborn mucus and relieve other symptoms that accompany coughs and colds, such as runny nose, catarrh, nasal congestion and blocked sinuses. Contains an antihistamine, triprolidine hydrochloride; a decongestant,

pseudoephedrine hydrochloride; and an expectorant, guaiphenesin. May cause drowsiness.

Dosage: As for Actifed Compound Linctus, above. As with all medicines, if you're pregnant or currently taking any other medicine, consult your doctor or pharmacist before taking this product.

WELLCOME

## Actifed Syrup and Actifed Tablets

A syrup or tablets to help soothe and relieve cold and flu symptoms such as stuffed-up nose, catarrh, runny nose and blocked sinuses. Also relieves summer cold and hay-fever symptoms, including sneezing, watery eyes, congested nasal passages and a runny nose. Contains an antihistamine, triprolidine hydrochloride, and a decongestant, pseudo-ephedrine hydrochloride. May cause drowsiness. As with all medicines, if you're pregnant or currently taking any other medicine, consult your doctor or pharmacist before taking this product.

Dosage – syrup: as for Actifed Expectorant, above. Dosage – tablets: adults and children over 12 only – one tablet three times a day.

WELLCOME

## Actron

A soluble, effervescent painkiller containing aspirin, paracetamol and caffeine for the relief of headaches, colds, influenza, feverishness, rheumatic and muscular pains, period pains, neuralgia and toothache. Not for children under 12. Dosage: two tablets every four hours, if necessary. No more than eight tablets in 24 hours.             BAYER CONSUMER

## Adult Kao-C and Junior Kao-C

Suspension flavoured with cinnamon, nutmeg and clove oils, containing light kaolin – a bulk-forming and absorbent agent, and calcium carbonate, an antacid, to calm the stomach for the treatment of short-term, mild diarrhoea. Adult Kao-C dosage: adults and children over 14 – four 5 ml spoonfuls three times a day. Junior Kao-C dosage: children over l4 – four 5 ml spoonfuls three times a day; 5–14 years – two 5 ml spoonfuls; 1–5 years – one 5 ml spoonful.             CUPAL

## Aezodent

A mildly anaesthetic ointment containing local pain-relievers benzocaine, chlorbutol and methyl salicylate, with analgesic, healing and antiseptic properties. Also contains eugenol and menthol. Used to combat chafing from dentures. Before inserting the denture in the mouth, squeeze a series of spots of the ointment on the denture, particularly where chafing is likely to occur.

ASSOCIATED DENTAL PRODUCTS

## Afrazine Nose Drops

To relieve stuffy noses for up to 12 hours. Contain the decongestant oxymetazoline hydrochloride. Dosage: adults and children over 5 years – two to three drops to be instilled into each nostril in the morning and at bedtime. For children under 5 use Afrazine Paediatric Nose Drops.             KIRBY-WARRICK

## Agarol

An emulsion for the temporary relief of constipation only. Particularly useful when it's not advisable to strain when opening the bowels – for those with a hernia, or convalescing after surgery, for example. Not suitable for children under 5. Contains phenolpthalein, liquid paraffin and agar, a carbohydrate obtained from seaweeds and used as a laxative. Adult dosage: one to three 5 ml spoonfuls to be taken at bedtime. If necessary, the dose may be repeated two

hours after breakfast.
Children 5–12 years – one 5
ml spoonful at bedtime or two
hours after breakfast. Agarol
may be mixed with water,
milk or fruit juices.

WARNER LAMBERT

## Algipan Rub

A non-greasy cream to bring
relief from muscular pain and
stiffness, especially in back
ache, sciatica, lumbago,
fibrositis and rheumatic pain.
Also available as a spray.
Contains methyl nicotinate,
which is used to make skin
redden and is therefore warm;
capiscin made from chillies;
and glycol salicylate, a
member of the aspirin family
used in rheumatic rubs.
Massage Algipan lightly into
the affected part until it's
completely absorbed into the
skin. Repeat two or three
times a day. Don't apply to
broken skin or near the eyes
or nose. Wash hands after
use.                    WYETH FAMILY HEALTH

## Alka-Seltzer

Effervescent tablets
containing aspirin, and, when
mixed with water, the
antacids sodium citrate and
sodium bicarbonate, for the
relief of headache with upset
stomach, particularly when
due to too much to eat or
drink. Alka-Seltzer is
especially effective when

taken before bed and again in
the morning. Can also be
taken for the relief of
migraine, period pain and
aches and pains associated
with colds and flu. Not
suitable for children under 12.

Dosage: two tablets in
water. The dose may be
repeated every four hours, up
to four doses in 24 hours.

BAYER CONSUMER

## Aller.eze

Tablets for relief from hay-
fever symptoms, itchy, watery
eyes, perennial rhinitis, insect
bites and skin allergies.
Contains the antihistamine
clemastine hydrogen
fumarate. Brings relief
without drowsiness in 90% of
users, but may cause
drowsiness in remaining 10%.
Not to be taken during
pregnancy or breast-feeding
except under medical
direction.

Dosage: adults and children
over 12 – one tablet night and
morning. Children 7–12 years
– half to one tablet night and
morning; 3–6 years – half a
tablet night and morning.
Tablets should be taken with
water before meals. Available
in elixir form for children
3–12 years.            INTERCARE

## Aller.eze Plus

Brings relief from nasal and

sinus congestion, hay fever and other allergy symptoms without drowsiness for 90% of users, but may cause drowsiness. Contains an antihistamine, clemastine hydrogen fumarate, and a decongestant, phenyl-propanolamine hydrochloride. Not recommended for children. Not to be taken during pregnancy or when breast-feeding.

Dosage: one tablet every six hours. No more than four tablets a day.          INTERCARE

## Alophen

Pills for the relief of constipation due to sluggishness of the lower bowel containing aloin, an irritant laxative; belladonna extract, a muscle relaxant; ipecacuanha root, used as a laxative; and phenolpthalein. Not suitable for children. Adults should take one to three pills at bedtime. Relief is usually prompt, occurring within eight to ten hours. Prolonged, continuous use is not recommended.

Alophen should not be used without a doctor's advice when nausea, vomiting or abdominal pain are present. It shouldn't be used by patients with inflammatory bowel diseases or with glaucoma, and should be used with

caution in patients with prostatic enlargement.
                    WARNER LAMBERT

## Aludrox

Tablets for the relief of indigestion, heartburn and acidity, containing aluminium hydroxide/magnesium carbonate co-dried gel and magnesium hydroxide. One or two tablets should be sucked or chewed four times daily and at bedtime, or as required.
          CHARWELL PHARMACEUTICALS

## Aludrox Liquid

Antacid liquid containing aluminium hydroxide, for the relief of indigestion, heartburn and acidity. Take one or two 5 ml spoonfuls undiluted or with a little water, either four times daily and at bedtime, or as required.
          CHARWELL PHARMACEUTICALS

## Anadin

Analgesic tablets, containing aspirin, caffeine and quinine sulphate, for relief of headache, neuralgia, colds and flu, rheumatic pain, period pain and dental pain. Not suitable for children under 12. Take two tablets every four hours, but no more than 12 tablets in any 24 hours. Also available in soluble form (soluble tablets do not contain quinine sulphate).          WHITEHALL

## Anadin Extra

Easy-to-swallow tablets, containing aspirin, paracetamol and caffeine, for the treatment of headache, migraine, neuralgia, rheumatic, period and dental pains and the symptoms of colds and influenza. Not suitable for children under 12.

Dosage: one or two tablets every four hours. No more than six tablets in any 24 hours.                    WHITEHALL

## Anadin Maximum Strength

Analgesic capsules containing aspirin and caffeine for the treatment of headache, migraine, neuralgia, rheumatic, period and dental pains and the symptoms of colds and flu. Not for children under 12.

Dosage: one to two capsules every four hours. No more than eight capsules in any 24 hours.                    WHITEHALL

## Anadin Paracetamol

Easy-to-swallow paracetamol tablets for the treatment of headache, migraine, neuralgia, rheumatic, period and dental pains and the symptoms of colds and flu. Not for children under six.

Dosage: adults and children over 12 – two tablets. Children 6–12 years – one tablet. The dose should not be repeated more frequently than every four hours and not more than four doses should be given in any 24-hour period.                    WHITEHALL

## Anbesol

Sugar-free liquid for mouth ulcers, teething pains and denture irritation. It contains lidocaine hydrochloride, a local anaesthetic, and chlorocresol and cetylpyridinium, both antiseptics. Apply to the affected area with the fingertip. Two applications immediately will normally be sufficient to obtain pain relief. Repeat as often as necessary. For teething in babies: wet the fingertip with Anbesol and spread gently on to the sore area of the gum. One application will be sufficient. Don't repeat the application for at least half an hour.

WHITEHALL

## Andrews Answer

An effervescent, lemon-flavoured drink to relieve headache with upset stomach. Contains a full 1 gm dose of paracetamol, so don't take other pain-relievers within four hours. Also contains the stimulant caffeine; an antacid, sodium bicarbonate, to settle the stomach; and citric acid, used as a flavouring.

Each sachet contains a complete dose. Dissolve the contents of one sachet in a glass of water, stir and drink when effervescence subsides. Don't take more than four sachets in 24 hours. Not suitable for children under 16.

STERLING HEALTH

## Andrews Liver Salt

A sparkling drink containing an antacid, sodium bicarbonate, and a laxative, magnesium sulphate (Epsom Salts), as well as sucrose and citric acid flavouring. Drink freshens the mouth, settles the stomach and revives the system. Can be used as an antacid to settle an upset stomach, relieve indigestion and biliousness, or as a laxative.

Dosage: adults only – empty contents of sachet into glass of water and drink before fizziness subsides. As an antacid, or as a refreshing drink, use one sachet. As a laxative, use two sachets before breakfast or at bedtime.          STERLING HEALTH

## Andursil

Tablets or liquid for the relief of gastric upsets. Andursil contain the antacids aluminium hydroxide and magnesium carbonate, and

activated polymethylsiloxane to relieve flatulence.

Dosage: one or two tablets at a time, up to a maximum of eight tablets a day. Liquid – half to one 5 ml spoonful, three to four times a day.

CIBA CONSUMER

## Anethane Itch-Soothing Cream

Cream containing tetracaine hydrochloride, a local anaesthetic, to give prompt relief from insect bites, stings and nettle rash. Not for prolonged use and not suitable for infants under three. Smooth cream on to affected area. Repeat as needed two or three times daily.     EVANS MEDICAL

## Anodesyn

Triple-action ointment for piles, containing lignocaine hydrochloride, a local anaesthetic to relieve pain; ephedrine hydrochloride, a vasoconstrictor which narrows walls of blood vessels to reduce swelling; and allantoin, to promote healing.

To treat internal piles, attach the nozzle to the tube, squeeze tube until ointment starts to appear through the nozzle, then gently insert the nozzle into the rectum. Squeeze out the ointment while slowly withdrawing the nozzle. Use night and morning and after each bowel movement.

For external piles, wash the affected area with tepid water, dry and apply the ointment with gauze or lint. Repeat as required. CROOKES HEALTHCARE

### Anthisan
Cream containing mepyramine maleate, an antihistamine, to relieve pain, itching and inflammation in nettle rash and insect bites and stings. Rub gently into affected areas two or three times daily for up to three days or as directed by your pharmacist or doctor. Discontinue should skin sensitivity occur. This cream should not be used for eczema or on extensively broken skin surfaces. If symptoms persist, consult your doctor. MAY & BAKER

### Antiseptic Throat Pastilles
Contain menthol, camphor and benzoic acid (an antiseptic) to soothe a dry, sore throat. Dissolve a pastille in the mouth as often as needed. ERNEST JACKSON

### Anusol
Suppositories, cream and ointment for the relief of piles and other related ano-rectal conditions. Contain the antiseptic Balsam Peru; protective substances bismuth oxide and zinc oxide; the suppositories and ointment also contain bismuth subgallate, which has astringent properties. Said to be safe for use during pregnancy, but always consult your doctor first.

Anusol should be used night and morning and after each bowel movement. The cream is also helpful as a lubricant for use with the suppositories. The ointment should be applied on a gauze dressing. WARNER LAMBERT

### APS Aspirin and Dispersible Aspirin Tablets
For the relief of pain and/or inflammation in headache, toothache, sore throat, feverish colds, influenza, period pain, sprains, strains, muscular aches and pains, lumbago, sciatica, fibrositis, rheumatism, joint swelling and stiffness.

Dosage: adults and children over 12 – one to three tablets every four hours (or less frequently) up to four times a day. Do not exceed 12 tablets in 24 hours. Dispersible tablets should be dissolved in water. APS

### Arret
Capsules for treatment of diarrhoea, containing loperamide hydrochloride

which slows down gut wall muscles. Not suitable for children under 12. Adults should take two capsules initially and one capsule after every loose bowel movement. The usual dosage is three to four capsules a day (maximum eight daily). JANSSEN PHARMACEUTICAL

## Asilone Tablets

For the relief of indigestion, acidity and heartburn, with dried aluminium hydroxide to combat excess acid and activated dimethicone to break down gas and relieve discomfort. Asilone gently soothes the stomach lining. Not suitable for children under 12. Dosage: one or two tablets chewed or sucked before meals and at bedtime. For the relief of heartburn, the tablets should be sucked slowly. Also available in liquid form – the liquid also contains the antacid light magnesium oxide. CROOKES HEALTHCARE

## Aspro

Tablets containing aspirin for the relief of headache, rheumatic pain, sore throats, colds, flu, muscular aches, neuralgia, period pain, toothache, lumbago, sciatica and fibrositis. Dosage: adults only – two to three tablets every four hours as needed.

No more than 12 tablets in 24 hours. NICHOLAS

## Aspro Clear and Aspro Clear Extra

Soluble tablets containing aspirin for the relief of headache, migraine pain, neuralgia, colds, chills, flu, fibrositis, period pain, muscular pain, toothache, rheumatic pain. Aspro Clear Extra can also be used for relief of lumbago and sciatica.

Dosage: Aspro Clear – two to three tablets dissolved in half a glass of water every four hours as needed. No more than 13 tablets in 24 hours. Aspro Clear Extra – one or two tablets dissolved in half a glass of water every four hours. No more than eight tablets in 24 hours.

NICHOLAS

## Avena Sativa Comp.

A calming homoeopathic remedy to help you relax at night after the stresses and strains of a difficult day. With *Avena sativa, Humulus lupulus, Passiflora incarnata,* valeriana, radix, *Coffea tosta.* Ten to 20 drops to be taken in water half an hour before retiring. If necessary, this dose may be repeated up to a maximum of six doses a day. Children should take half the adult dose. WELEDA

### Bath E45

Dermatological bath oil to soothe and soften dry skin conditions, containing medicinal white oil to soften skin and cetyl dimethicone which acts as a barrier to protect against the irritating and drying effects of water or detergents.

Pour quarter of a capful into warm water, or apply on a wet sponge when showering. Blot skin gently with towel. Take care not to slip and, as with soap, avoid contact with the eyes.

CROOKES HEALTHCARE

### Bayer Aspirin

Tablets containing acetylsalicylic acid (aspirin) for the relief of headache, colds and rheumatic pains.

Dosage: adults – one to three tablets with water, up to four times a day, at four-hourly intervals if necessary. No more than 12 tablets in 24 hours.                 BAYER

### Benoxyl 5 or 10 and Benoxyl Creams with Sulphur

Grease-free antiseptic medications containing benzoyl peroxide for treatment of acne. Apply daily. Also available in lotion form. Where it is present, the sulphur acts as a mild antiseptic.                 STIEFEL

### Bengue's Balsam

Topical rubefacient with menthol and methyl salicylate for easing pain due to rheumatic conditions and muscular strain. Massage up to four times a day. Can also be used as an inhalation from hot water for the symptomatic relief of congestion associated with head colds. Can be used to relieve chilblains but only on unbroken skin. Available in two strengths.

SYNTEX PHARMACEUTICALS

### Benylin

A syrup for the relief of coughs and the symptoms associated with phlegm. Works by dampening the cough and suppresses the production of phlegm to stop the runny nose. Contains an antihistamine, diphen-hydramine hydrochloride, and soothing menthol. Diphenhydramine hydro-chloride can help relieve coughs because its antitussive – cough-suppressant – and antihistaminic action neutralises the effects of histamine released by the body in allergic reactions. Benylin's anticholinergic actions block nerve impulses, especially those used to control intestinal spasm. It helps provide relief from nasal stuffiness, sneezing and watering of the eyes. It also has a local anaesthetic action which helps to relieve sore throats. May cause drowsiness. Can be taken by children, although for children from 1–4 years, Benylin Paediatric is recommended. Children from 6–12 years should take one 5 ml spoonful four times a day. Adult dosage: two 5 ml spoonfuls four times a day. WARNER LAMBERT

## Benylin with Codeine

Cough syrup for dry, irritating coughs. Combines the antitussive, antihistaminic, local anaesthetic and anticholinergic effects of diphenhydramine hydrochloride with the suppressive action of codeine phosphate. Also contains menthol. May cause drowsiness. Codeine may be habit-forming. Not recommended for children under five. Children 6–12 should take one 5 ml spoonful four times a day. Adult dosage: two 5 ml spoonfuls four times a day. WARNER LAMBERT

## Benylin Children's Cough Linctus

To give relief to the coughing child and to reduce bronchial and nasal congestion. Also beneficial in the treatment of

hay fever and other allergic conditions affecting the upper respiratory tract. Combines the actions of diphen-hydramine hydrochloride (see BENYLIN, above) with the demulcent agent menthol, a soothing substance to help combat the congestive symptoms that frequently accompany the cough and reduce bronchial and nasal congestion. Not recommended for children under one year old. Dosage: children 6–12 years, two 5 ml spoonfuls four times a day; 1–5 years – one 5 ml spoonful four times a day. May cause drowsiness. WARNER LAMBERT

## Benylin Day and Night Cold Treatment

A blister pack with 15 amber film-coated tablets and five blue film-coated tablets for the relief of symptoms associated with colds and flu. Amber tablets (daytime) combine the analgesic and antipyretic (fever-reducing) action of paracetamol with the decongestant action of phenyl-propanolamine hydrochloride. Blue (night-time) tablets combine paracetamol with the antihistamine, antitussive, antispasmodic and sedative action of diphenhydramine hydrochloride. May cause drowsiness. Not to be used in pregnancy. Not recommended for children under 12.

Dosage: four tablets daily, three amber during the day and one blue at night. Take only one tablet at a time and only at the times of day indicated on the pack. Do not take the night-time tablets during the day.   WARNER LAMBERT

## Benylin Dry Cough Linctus

Contains diphenhydramine hydrochloride (see BENYLIN, above) to control dry, irritating coughs and the cough-suppressant dextromethorphan hydrobromide. Also contains menthol. Adult dosage: two 5 ml spoonfuls four times a day. Children 6–12 years – one 5 ml spoonful four times a day. For one to five-year-olds, Benylin Children's Cough Linctus is recommended (see above). Not recommended for children under one year old. May cause drowsiness.

WARNER LAMBERT

## Benylin Mentholated Linctus

Menthol-tasting and -smelling linctus to relieve nasal stuffiness, sneezing, watering of the eyes and sore throats. Particularly suitable for coughs associated with colds. Contains diphenhydramine

hydrochloride (see BENYLIN, above), dextromethorphan hydrobromide to suppress the cough reflex and pseudo-ephedrine hydrochloride to combat the congestive symptoms that frequently accompany the cough and to reduce bronchial and nasal congestion.

Dosage: adults – two 5 ml spoonfuls four times daily. Children 6–12 years – one 5 ml spoonful four times daily. May cause drowsiness.

WARNER LAMBERT

## Benzagel 5 and 10

Gels containing benzoyl peroxide for the treatment of acne. Start treatment with Benzagel 5. Wash the affected areas with soap and water (this helps the Benzagel to penetrate the skin), dry and apply gel once or twice daily. The therapeutic response to benzoyl peroxide differs in individual patients, so you may need to use the stronger Benzagel 10.

BIOGLAN PHARMACEUTICALS

## Biactol

Face wash with phenyoxylpropanol, an antibacterial, in a mild detergent base. Suitable for sensitive skin. Use daily instead of soap.

PROCTER AND GAMBLE

## Bidor 1% Tablets

A course of treatment containing ferrous sulphate monohydrate and silica for the prevention of migraine. One tablet should be taken three times a day to help prevent the development of migraine attacks. Continue treatment for a period of from two to 12 weeks, according to the severity of the condition, to reduce the tendency to attacks. Bidor tablets should be swallowed with water, not chewed.                    WELEDA

## Bioral Gel

Contains carbenoxolone sodium for the treatment of mouth ulcers. Carbenoxolone is thought to help soothe ulcers by provoking protective mucus production. Pat ulcer dry with a tissue and cover with a thick coating of Bioral. Apply after meals and at bedtime. Suitable for both adults and children.

STERLING HEALTH

## Bismag Tablets

Antacid tablets for the relief of indigestion, flatulence and stomach acidity, containing sodium bicarbonate and heavy and light magnesium carbonate. Take two to four tablets with water after meals and repeat in 15 minutes if

necessary. A dose before going to bed is recommended.

WHITEHALL

## BiSoDol Extra

Antacid tablets for the relief of heartburn, indigestion, acidity and flatulence, containing calcium carbonate, light magnesium carbonate, sodium bicarbonate and simethicone to break down gas. Take one or two tablets as required. Suck slowly or chew.                    WHITEHALL

## BiSoDol Powder

Mint-flavoured antacid powder for the relief of indigestion, dyspepsia, heartburn, acidity and flatulence. It contains sodium bicarbonate and heavy and light magnesium carbonate.

Dosage: one 5 ml spoonful well stirred into about one third of a tumbler of water (warm or cold) after meals or as required.                    WHITEHALL

## BiSoDol Tablets

Antacid digestant tablets for the relief of indigestion, dyspepsia, heartburn, acidity and flatulence. They contain calcium carbonate, light magnesium carbonate and sodium bicarbonate. Take one or two tablets, as required. Suck slowly or chew.    WHITEHALL

### Blistex

Soothing lip balm with sun protection factor, sunscreens padimate and oxybenzone and protective agent dimethicone; also contains other emollients, including cocoa butter and lanolin, to soften dry, chapped lips. Apply as required.   BLISTEX

### Blisteze Cream

For the quick relief of occasional cold sores, cracked and chapped lips. Contains a strong ammonia solution, an aromatic intended to relieve pain, and liquefied phenol, an antiseptic. Apply as soon as symptoms appear and repeat every hour if necessary. If you suffer from recurrent cold sores, consult your doctor.

BLISTEX

### Bocasan Mouthwash

Bocasan is buffered sodium perborate monohydrate, an oxygenating oral rinse which supplies oxygen for the inhibition of the action of bacteria. It's also antiseptic and cleansing, used for the treatment of bleeding gums and other symptoms of gum disease and helpful in the control of dental plaque. Bocasan is suitable for use by both adults and children over five, although care should be taken to prevent children from swallowing the solution.

Use three times daily after meals. Dissolve the contents of one sachet in 30 ml of warm water – as hot as you would normally drink a cup of tea – and use immediately. Hold the rinse in the mouth for two to three minutes, swishing between the teeth. Do not swallow. After rinsing with Bocasan, do not cleanse the mouth with any other liquid for 30 minutes. Don't use for longer than seven days without consulting your doctor or dentist.   ORAL-B

### Bonomint

Mint-flavoured chewing gum laxative with yellow phenophthalein. For overnight relief, chew before going to bed. It is only necessary to chew a tablet until the flavour is gone. Do not swallow.

Dosage: adults – one to two tablets; children over 6 – half to one tablet.   INTERCARE

### Bradosol and Bradosol Plus

Throat lozenges containing the antiseptic domiphen bromide for the relief of sore throats. Bradosol Plus also contains the local anaesthetic lignocaine hydrochloride to numb sore throats and fight infection.   CIBA CONSUMER

## Brasivol Fine

Cleanser for acne containing scrub particles of fused aluminium oxide, an abrasive to clean the skin thoroughly. Before using, discontinue the use of all other soaps and skin cleansers. Apply to wet skin, rubbing gently in a circular motion for 15–20 seconds. Rinse with warm water and pat dry. Repeat two to three times daily or as directed by your doctor. If undue skin irritation occurs, discontinue use and consult your doctor.

STIEFEL

## Bronal Cough Balsam

Contains dextromethorphan hydrobromide, a cough-suppressant, and soothing glycerin for the relief of dry, ticklish, unproductive coughs in adults and children over 12. May cause slight drowsiness.

Dosage: one 5 ml spoonful three times a day.          CUPAL

## Bronalin Dry Cough Elixir

Sugar- and colour-free elixir for the symptomatic relief of dry, tickly coughs and colds. Contains the cough-suppressant dextro-methorphan hydrobromide and pseudoephedrine hydro-chloride to fight congestion. Recommended for use by those with diabetes, but not for children under six.

Asthmatics should consult their doctor before using this product. May cause drowsiness.

Dosage: adults – one 5 ml spoonful four times a day; children 6–12 years – half a 5 ml spoonful four times a day.

CUPAL

## Bronalin Expectorant Linctus

Sugar- and colour-free linctus containing the expectorants ammonium chloride and sodium citrate, and diphenhydramine hydrochloride, an antihistamine, for the symptomatic relief of deep, chesty coughs and colds. May cause drowsiness. Not for children under six. Not to be taken during pregnancy.

Dosage, to be taken three or four times daily: adults – one or two 5 ml spoonfuls; children 6–12 years, one 5 ml spoonful.          CUPAL

## Bronalin Paediatric Linctus

Sugar-free, blackcurrant-flavoured linctus for the symptomatic relief of children's coughs and colds. Contains sodium citrate, an expectorant, and diphen-hydramine hydrochloride, an antihistamine. May cause drowsiness. Recommended for use by those suffering from diabetes.

Dosage, to be taken three times daily: children 5–12 years – two 5 ml spoonfuls; 1–5 years one 5 ml spoonful.

CUPAL

## Bronchial Catarrh Pastilles

Contain soothing menthol, benzoin tincture, creosote (a disinfectant), aniseed oil, peppermint oil and capiscin (made from peppers) to relieve bronchial catarrh, coughs and colds.

ERNEST JACKSON

## Brooklax

Chocolate-flavoured laxative tablets with yellow phenolphthalein to relieve constipation. Should ideally be taken before going to bed.

Dosage: adults – half to two tablets; children over 6 – a quarter to one tablet.

INTERCARE

## Burn Aid Cream

Soothing cream containing aminacrine hydrochloride, an antiseptic, for first-aid treatment of minor burns and scalds, cuts and abrasions. Apply to sore area and cover with a dressing if appropriate. Do not use repeatedly. Prolonged use may delay healing.

CUPAL

## Burneze

First-aid spray for minor burns and scalds, containing the local anaesthetic benzocaine. If the burn is extensive, seek medical help immediately. To reduce pain and blistering, use spray as quickly as possible. Spray 0.5 cm ($\frac{1}{4}$ in) from skin until all the pain has gone – this may take up to five seconds. If white frost appears, stop. Repeat after 15 minutes if necessary. Do not apply lint, bandage or other dressing. Don't spray near eyes, and don't apply to broken skin.

INTERNATIONAL LABORATORIES

## Cal-A-Cool

Soothing cream containing calamine and skin protective agents zinc oxide and dimethicone. Apply freely to the affected parts.

CUPAL

## Caladryl

Soothing cream or lotion for the relief of irritation associated with hives, shingles and other minor skin complaints. Also helpful in the relief of sunburn, prickly heat, insect bites and nettle stings. Contains protective agent zinc oxide, antihistamine diphenyhdramine hydrochloride and cooling camphor.

The lotion can be dabbed on the affected skin using a pad of cotton wool. The cream can be smoothed on lightly. But Caladryl shouldn't be put on raw skin or mucous membranes. If a burning sensation or rash develops, or if the condition persists, treatment should be discontinued.                WARNER LAMBERT

## Calendula Lotion

A healing lotion containing calendula for cuts, abrasions or minor wounds and skin infections. May be used as a mouthwash. Add one 5 ml spoonful to a glass of cooled boiled water to cleanse wound or to use as a compress; one 5 ml spoonful to half a glass of lukewarm boiled water for a mouthwash.                WELEDA

## Califig

California Syrup of Figs with senna, a natural irritant laxative, for relief from constipation for all the family. To be taken at bedtime.

Dosage: adults – one to two 15 ml spoonfuls. Children 6–15 years – one and a half to three 5 ml spoonfuls; 3–6 years – one to two 5 ml spoonfuls; 1–3 years – half to one 5 ml spoonful.
                STERLING HEALTH

## Calgel

A sugar-free gel for teething pain, containing lignocaine hydrochloride and cetylpyridiunium chloride. Repeat after 20 minutes if necessary, up to six times in one day.                WELLCOME

## Calpol Infant Suspension

Paracetamol suspension to relieve pain, including teething pain and feverishness such as accompanies colds and flu, without irritating the stomach. Most suitable for babies and children from three months to six years. Also available in sugar-free form.

Dosage: children 1–6 years – one to two 5 ml spoonfuls; babies 3 months to 1 year – half to one 5 ml spoonful. Under three months, on doctor's advice only. Don't give more than four doses in 24 hours. Don't repeat doses more frequently than every four hours, and don't continue treatment for more than three days without consulting a doctor.                WELLCOME

## Calpol Six Plus

Paracetamol suspension for pain associated with headaches, toothache and fever relief for children over six years old.

Dosage, to be taken four times a day: adults and

children over 12 – two to four
5ml spoonfuls. Children 6–12
years – one to two 5 ml
spoonfuls. For children three
months to under six years,
Calpol Infant Suspension is
recommended (see above).
The safety advice given for
Calpol Infant Suspension also
applies to this product. WELLCOME

## Capasal Therapeutic Shampoo

For the treatment of dandruff,
scalp psoriasis, seborrhoeic
dermatitis and cradle cap.
Contains salicylic acid, whose
keratolytic action loosens and
removes scalp scale and scalp
debris; coconut oil, an
effective emollient to soften
and moisturise the scalp; and
coal tar, an antipruritic (itch-
soothing) and therapeutic
agent. Use as a shampoo, daily
if necessary. Leave lather on
for a few minutes before
washing out. Apparently safe
for use in pregnancy and for
children – there are no known
side-effects in either case.

DERMAL LABORATORIES

## Carnation Corn Caps

Corn caps with a ring of felt
to relieve pressure on the corn
and give immediate relief.
Also contain salicylic acid to
reduce the size of the corn.
Packs contain five corn caps
for a ten-day treatment.

CUXSON GERRARD

## Catarrh-Ex

Tablets with paracetamol and
the decongestant pseudo-
ephedrine hydrochloride for
the relief of congestion
associated with pain and fever.
Relieves the symptoms of
nasal congestion, blocked
sinuses, feverishness, aches,
pains, colds and flu.

Dosage, to be taken three
times a day: adults and
children over 12 – one tablet.
Children 6–12 years – half a
tablet.                    JEFFREY MARTIN

## Catarrh Pastilles

Contain soothing menthol,
abietis pine oil, sylvestris pine
oil and creosote (a
disinfectant) to ease the
symptoms of catarrh and an
irritating cough. Dissolve one
pastille slowly in the mouth
when required.      ERNEST JACKSON

## Cepton

Skin wash, lotion and gel for
the treatment of acne,
containing chlorhexidine
gluconate, an antiseptic.

CIBA CONSUMER

## Cerumol

Ear drops for the loosening
and removal of ear wax. They
contain paradichlorobenzene,
an insecticide, chlorbutol,
which has antibacterial
properties, and arachis oil.
Insert five drops into the ear
when the head is inclined,

preferably when lying down. This may cause a harmless tingling sensation. If the drops run out when the head is held up, a small plug of cotton wool moistened with Cerumol may be applied. Repeat two or three times daily for up to three days. Unless the ear wax is unusually hard it should run out of its own accord. If not, consult your doctor for possible syringing. You are advised to consult your doctor in all cases of ear disorder before using any ear drops. Use this product within six months of opening.

LABORATORIES FOR APPLIED BIOILOGY

## Chamomilla 3 × Drops or Pillules

Third homoeopathic potency of *Matricaria chamomilla* for the relief of colicky pain and teething troubles in infants.

Dosage – drops: five to ten drops to be taken in a little water three times a day, or, if necessary, five drops can be taken every half hour until the condition improves, for up to four hours. Dosage – pilules: one to five pilules to be dissolved in the mouth every half hour until the condition improves. For children under six months, the pilules may be crushed.

WELEDA

## Chilblain Cream

Cream containing methyl nicotinate, a vasodilator – it helps bring blood to the surface of the skin and can help improve circulation, for the symptomatic relief of aches associated with chilblains. Gently bathe affected parts in warm water. Dry carefully. Apply cream sparingly morning and night and more frequently if needed.          J. PICKLES & SONS

## Children's Cough Pastilles

Contain honey, ascorbic acid, squill liquid extract and ipecacuanha liquid extract – expectorants, to ease a child's persistent cough. Pastilles can be taken as needed, but limited over a 24-hour period as follows: children over 8 years – 12 pastilles; 6–8 years – ten pastilles; 3–5 years – eight pastilles.     ERNEST JACKSON

## Cirkulin Garlic Pearls

Contain organically grown Chinese garlic. May help relieve colds and maintain a healthy heart and circulation. Take two tablets three times a day with a little water, ideally before meals. Swallow whole.

CEDAR HEALTH

## Clearasil Medicated Cleansing Milk and Lotion

Antibacterial cleansing milk for combination skin and lotion for oily skin to help prevent spots. Wash face and neck with a mild soap, moisten cotton pad with lotion or milk and cleanse. Repeat with fresh cotton pads until no trace of dirt remains. Do not rinse once cleansing is complete. Use morning and night.           PROCTER AND GAMBLE

## Clearasil Medicated Cream

For treatment of spots and blackheads. Contains triclosan, an antibacterial agent, and precipitated sulphur, an antiseptic; it works by killing the bacteria that can cause spots. Ultra Clearasil, with benzoyl peroxide, is also available. Spread over problem areas, or directly on to spots.
                    PROCTER AND GAMBLE

## Clearasil Medicated Gel

Contains salicylic acid for treatment of spots and blackheads. Spread over problem areas night and morning.           PROCTER AND GAMBLE

## Coda-Med

Tablets with paracetamol, codeine phosphate and caffeine for the symptomatic relief of tension headache, rheumatic pain, toothache, neuralgia, period pain, flu and colds. Also help to lower the temperature in mild feverish conditions. Not to be given to children under eight except on medical advice. No more than four doses to be taken in 24 hours.

Dosage: adults – one or two tablets every four hours. Children 8–14 years – one tablet every four hours.
                    JEFFREY MARTIN

## Codanin

Strong analgesic tablets containing paracetamol and codeine for the relief of bad headaches, migraine, period pains, neuralgia, rheumatic pains and dental pain. Not suitable for children under six except on medical advice.

Dosage: adults – two tablets with water at three- to four-hour intervals as required. Don't exceed eight tablets in 24 hours. Children 6-12 years – half a tablet with water as above. Don't exceed four doses in 24 hours.           WHITEHALL

## Codis 500

Analgesic tablets containing aspirin and codeine phosphate for the relief of mild to moderate pain including headache, migraine, neuralgia, toothache, period pains, aches and pains and the symptoms of colds, influenza and feverish conditions. Also for the symptomatic relief of sprains, strains, rheumatic pain, sciatica, lumbago, fibrositis, muscular aches and pains, joint swelling and stiffness.

Dosage – adults and children over 12: one to two tablets as directed, dissolved in water. The dose may be repeated after four hours. Maximum eight tablets in 24 hours in divided doses. Not for children under 12 except on doctor's advice.

RECKITT & COLMAN

## Coldrex
Available as tablets, blackcurrant-flavoured drink or real lemon-flavoured drink, for relief from the symptoms of colds and flu, and to soothe sore throats. Tablets contain paracetamol; phenylephrine hydrochloride to clear a stuffy nose; the stimulant caffeine; terpin hydrate, a cough expectorant; and Vitamin C. Drinks do not contain expectorant or caffeine. Take tablets at first signs of a cold or flu every four hours.

Dosage – tablets: adults – two tablets up to four times a day. Children 6–12 years – one tablet up to four times a day. Not to be given to children under six. Dosage: adults – one sachet up to four times a day. Empty contents

into a tumbler and fill with very hot water. Stir until dissolved and sweeten if desired with honey or sugar. Not to be given to children under 12.

Some medicines don't combine with these products. If you are pregnant or already taking medicines, ask your doctor's advice before taking Coldrex. STERLING HEALTH

## J. Collis Browne's Tablets
Peppermint-flavoured tablets containing light kaolin, morphine hydrochloride and calcium carbonate to treat diarrhoea in colic, mild forms of gastro-enteritis, mild food poisoning and 'holiday tummy'. Not suitable for children under six.

Dosage: adults and children over 10 – two to three tablets at once, followed by two to three tablets every four hours. Chew tablets before swallowing. Children 6-10 years, one tablet at once, followed by one tablet every four hours.

INTERNATIONAL LABORATORIES

## J. Collis Browne's Mixture
For the relief of diarrhoea and tummy upsets. Contains anhydrous morphine to slow down the movement of the bowel wall.

Dosage: adults and children

over 12 – two to three 5 ml spoonfuls once or twice at four-hourly intervals if required. Children 6–12 years – one 5 ml spoonful as above. Not suitable for children under six.

INTERNATIONAL LABORATORIES

## Combudoron Lotion

Homoepathic lotion with extracts of *Urtica urens*, Herba, *Arnica montana* and *Planta tota*, for the relief of sunburn, insect bites, minor burns and minor rashes, including nettle rash. Use one 5 ml spoonful to a cup of boiled water. Soak a piece of lint in the solution and apply as a compress. Keep moist. Use the lotion undiluted on insect bites.

WELEDA

## Compound W

Liquid wart- and verruca-remover containing salicylic acid. Not to be used for children under six. Apply a drop at a time until the wart or verruca is covered. Cover with a waterproof plaster. Repeat daily for up to four weeks, removing and replacing or changing the plaster each day until the wart or verruca disappears.

WHITEHALL LABORATORIES

## Congesteze Syrup

All-round relief from blocked-up, runny nose and catarrh, containing pseudoephedrine sulphate, a decongestant to ease breathing and reduce painful nasal and sinus swelling, and azatadine maleate, an antihistamine to help dry up runny noses and stop sneezing. Also effective in the treatment of hay fever. May cause drowsiness.

Dosage: adults and children over 12 years – one 5 ml spoonful each morning and at bedtime. Children 6–12 years – half to one 5 ml spoonful each morning and at bedtime, or as directed by your doctor. Not to be taken by children under six. For children 1–6 years use Congesteze Paediatric Syrup, dosage one 5 ml spoonful in the morning and at bedtime.

KIRBY-WARRICK

## Conotrane

Medicated cream with dimethicone, a water-repellant, and benzalkonium chloride, a mild but effective antiseptic, for the treatment and prevention of nappy rash. Apply to the affected area several times a day as necessary or after every nappy change.

BOEHRINGER INGELHEIM

## Contac 400

Capsules containing phenylpropanolamine hydrochloride, which constricts blood vessels to ease congestion, and chlorpheniramine maleate, an antihistamine. Gives up to 12 hours' relief from cold and allergy symptoms such as runny nose, sneezing and congestion.                    WELLCOME

## Copholco

Cough syrup for the relief of ticklish coughs with pholcodine (a cough-suppressant), terpin hydrate (an expectorant), menthol and aromatic cineole.

Dosage: adults – two 5 ml spoonfuls without water to be sipped slowly four to five times daily. Children over 5 years – half to one 5 ml spoonful taken as above. As with any medicine, if you are pregnant or breast-feeding, consult your doctor before taking this product.         FISONS

## Copholcoids

Cough pastilles for the relief of ticklish coughs with the same active ingredient and safety advice as Copholco syrup, above. Adults should suck one or two pastilles three or four times daily according to the severity of the condition. Children over 5

years – suck one pastille three times daily at four-hourly intervals.                    FISONS

## Copper Ointment

For the relief of muscular rheumatic pain containing a copper salt in a base with yellow soft paraffin. Apply thinly and massage well into the affected area once or twice a day.                    WELEDA

## Correctol Laxative

Gentle laxative with dioctyl sodium sulphusuccinate to soften intestinal waste that has become too dry and hard, and yellow phenolphthalein, a laxative. Not to be used during pregnancy or breast-feeding. Not recommended for children under 12.

Dosage: adults and children over 12 – one tablet as needed at bedtime or on waking.
                    KIRBY-WARRICK

## Cradocap Shampoo

A gentle shampoo for the treatment of cradle cap, containing cetrimide, an antibacterial and cleanser which helps prevent infection, and lanolin to soften the scales and help remove them. Wet the baby's head, squeeze 2 cm of shampoo on to your hand and rub it in gently. Rinse off backwards to avoid contact with baby's eyes. Repeat and then dry. Do this twice a week until the condition clears.   NAPP

## Crampex

Tablets containing nicotinic acid – one of the Vitamin B group; calcium in the form of calcium gluconate; and cholecalciferol – Vitamin D3; for the relief of muscle cramp at night. Not recommended for children.

Dosage: adults, including the elderly – one or two tablets with a drink, preferably before retiring. If symptoms persist, consult your doctor.

INTERNATIONAL LABORATORIES

## Cream E45

Unperfumed, non-greasy, dermatological cream for dry skin conditions. Contains the emollients white soft paraffin, light liquid paraffin and anhydrous lanolin. Helpful in treatment of sunburn, flaking, chapped skin, nappy soreness, 'detergent hands', dermatitis, the dry stage of eczema and certain cases of psoriasis. Also helps soften rough, hard skin on other parts of the body.

CROOKES HEALTHCARE

## Cupal Baby Chest Rub

Menthol, eucalyptus and turpentine oil rub for babies and young children, for symptomatic relief of nasal catarrh and congestion due to colds. Rub on the chest, throat and back morning and night. Leave bedding and clothes loose to allow easy inhalation of the vapours. Don't apply directly to the nostrils and keep away from the eyes.

CUPAL

## Cupal Baby Cough Syrup

A blackcurrant-flavoured, sugar-free syrup to relieve and soothe the irritating and distressing coughs often accompanying colds. Specially prepared for babies over three months and young children, it contains dilute acetic acid, an expectorant.

Dosage, to be given slowly: three months to a year – half a 5 ml spoonful. Over 1 year – one 5 ml spoonful. Over $2\frac{1}{2}$ years – two 5 ml spoonfuls. Repeat as necessary every two or three hours.   CUPAL

## Cupal Cold Sore Lotion

Contains the antiseptic povidine iodine for the treatment of skin infections caused by bacteria and viruses, especially cold sores. Apply twice daily to the affected area and allow to dry. Avoid use in rare cases of iodine sensitivity.

CUPAL

## Cupal Cold Sore Ointment

Soothing antiseptic for the treatment of cold sores containing diperodon hydrochloride, a local anaesthetic; allantoin to encourage healing; cooling camphor; and protective zinc oxide. Apply the ointment to cold sores on the lips, five or six times a day.    CUPAL

## Cupal Corn Solvent and Pads

Corn-softening treatment containing salicylic acid. Apply liberally to top and side of corn. Allow to dry before covering foot. Repeat once or twice daily for four to seven days, then soak the foot in warm water and lift out the corn with a clean nail file or similar implement.    CUPAL

## Cupal Insect Bite Cream

For quick relief of wasp stings and other insect bites. Contains antazoline hydrochloride, an antihistamine. Apply to the affected area immediately after being stung. Repeat every 30 minutes if necessary.    CUPAL

## Cupal Wart Solvent

Contains glacial acetic acid for the removal of warts. Apply a small quantity to head of wart only, each morning and night for two or three weeks. Do not use on tender or broken warts.    CUPAL

## Cupal Verruca Treatment

Ointment containing salicylic acid, pads and plasters for the treatment of small, round verrucas. Cover verruca with pad. Put ointment on to verruca, cover with plaster and leave for two to three days. Repeat as necessary.    CUPAL

## Cupal Wax-Aid Ear Drops

Medicated drops containing turpentine and arachis oil to soften the wax; local pain-reliever and antibacterial agent chlorbutol; and paradichlorobenzene to relieve the symptoms associated with hardened wax in the ears and to aid its removal. Put three or four drops into the affected ear morning and night until the wax softens and can easily be removed with cotton wool.    CUPAL

## Cupanol Over Six

Sugar-free, colour-free, animal-fat-free paracetamol suspension for the relief of mild to moderate pain including headache, migraine, neuralgia, toothache and sore throat in children over six. Also for the symptomatic

relief of flu, feverishness and
colds.

Dose to be taken no more
frequently than every four
hours, and no more than four
doses in 24 hours. Adults and
children over 12 – two to four
5 ml spoonfuls. Children 6–12
– one to two 5 ml spoonfuls.

CUPAL

## Cupanol Under Six

Sugar-free, colour-free
paracetamol oral suspension
ᶠor the relief of pain and
feverish conditions in children
over three months old.

Dose to be taken four times
daily – don't repeat more
frequently than every four
hours. Children over 5 years –
three or four 5 ml spoonfuls.
Children 1–5 years – two 5 ml
spoonfuls. Three months to
one year, half to one 5 ml
spoonful.    CUPAL

## Cuprofen Ibuprofen Tablets

For the relief of headaches,
migraine, neuralgia and
fibrositis, backache and
lumbago, rheumatic and
muscular pains, period and
dental pains. Also for the
symptomatic relief of colds,
flu and feverishness. Not
suitable for children under 12.
Best taken after food.

Dosage: adults and children
over 12 – initial dose, two

tablets to be taken with water.
May be followed by further
doses of one or two tablets
every four hours. Do not
exceed six tablets in 24 hours.

CUPAL

## Cymalon

A 48-hour course of soluble
granules to relieve the
symptoms of cystitis.
Contains sodium citrate and
sodium bicarbonate to make
urine less acid. Also contains
citric acid.

Empty one sachet into a
glass of cold water. Stir until
dissolved, then drink. Take
one sachet in water three
times daily over 48 hours.
You should take all six sachets
to complete the treatment.

STERLING HEALTH

## Cystoleve

A 48-hour treatment for
cystitis containing sodium
citrate to make urine less acid.
Directions – as for Cymalon,
above.    CUPAL

## Cystopurin

A 48-hour course for relief of
cystitis, containing potassium
citrate to make urine less acid.
Take one sachet dissolved in
water three times daily over
48 hours. All six sachets must
be taken to complete the
course. Do not take
Cystopurin without first

consulting your doctor if you are pregnant or have had any kidney disease. Not for children under six.                    FISONS

## Daktarin Cream

Contains miconazole nitrate – an antifungal and antibacterial drug which destroys fungus and its spores. Used to treat minor fungal and some bacterial infections of the skin, such as athlete's foot, 'dhobie itch', intertrigo and infected nappy rash. Apply to affected area twice a day. Relief from symptoms may occur quickly, but it is important that you continue to use cream for up to ten days after the symptoms have cleared.

JANSSEN PHARMACEUTICAL

## Daktarin Oral Gel

Sugar-free gel containing miconazole (see Daktarin Cream, above) to treat fungal infections of the lips, mouth and throat such as oral thrush in babies and adults and due to denture chafing. Specially formulated to adhere to mucous membranes for up to six hours after application.

Dosage: adults and children over 6 – squeeze a small amount of gel on to a clean finger and apply to the affected area four times a day after food. Children under 6 – use twice a day. For oral thrush caused by denture chafing, it may be useful to smear a small amount of gel on to the denture plate. For best results, keep the gel in contact with the affected area for as long as possible before you have to swallow, and then swallow it. Relief from symptoms may occur quickly, but it's important that you continue to use gel for up to two days after the symptoms have cleared. If you are pregnant, consult your doctor before using the gel.

JANSSEN PHARMACEUTICAL

## Daktarin Powder

Medicated talc with miconazole (see Daktarin Cream, above) for the treatment of fungal infections such as infected nappy rash, intertrigo and athlete's foot. It is particularly useful where a drying effect is needed and may be used on broken skin. Apply to affected area twice daily. Also available in spray powder form to cool and soothe.            JANSSEN PHARMACEUTICAL

## Deep Heat-Deep Freeze Cold Gel

A menthol rub for tired muscles, after sports, gardening or exercise. Combines the benefits of muscle massage with the soothing sensation of coldness. Also helpful for rheumatic pain and stiff limbs and joints. Apply liberally to the required area. Massage until gel is completely absorbed into the skin. Use as needed. Also available in spray form for painful muscular spasms.   MENTHOLATUM

## Deep Heat Extra Strength Intensive Therapy

A soothing rub with menthol and the counter-irritant methyl salicylate, for the relief of nagging muscular aches and rheumatic pain. Not suitable for young children. Massage into affected area until penetration of the cream is complete. Apply two or three times daily.   MENTHOLATUM

## Deep Heat Extra Strength Pain-Relieving Lotion

Extra strong emulsion with menthol and the counter-irritant methyl salicylate for fast relief from the pain of rheumatism, fibrositis, lumbago, muscular aches, strains and stiffness caused by strenuous exercise. Not suitable for children under five. Massage affected area until lotion is absorbed. Repeat two or three times daily.   MENTHOLATUM

## Deep Heat Pre-Sport Rub

Contains menthol and methyl salicylate, a counter-irritant, to prime muscles for action before sport. Massage lotion firmly against muscles to warm up muscle fibres and help increase blood supply.

MENTHOLATUM

## Deep Heat Rub

A warming, pain-relieving rub to provide effective relief from rheumatic pain and all muscular aches, pains and strains. Contains soothing menthol, eucalyptus and turpentine oil, and the counter-irritant methyl salicylate, to stimulate the blood flow and relax stiffness. Massage into affected area until penetration of cream is complete.   MENTHOLATUM

## Denorex

Anti-dandruff shampoo to clear dandruff and soothe irritation, scaling, itching and flaking. Also suitable for treatment of psoriasis of the scalp and seborrhoeic dermatitis. Contains coal tar to stop itching and to moisturise, and soothing menthol. Apply every other day for first ten days (or daily if necessary), then two to three times a week until signs of dandruff disappear. Repeat once a week after that. Use as ordinary shampoo, but leave on the hair for two to three minutes.                    WHITEHALL

## Dentinox Cradle-Cap Shampoo

A treatment shampoo for infant cradle cap and general care of the scalp and hair. Contains sodium lauryl ether sulpho-succinate and sodium lauryl ether sulphate, both medicated cleansers. Wet baby's head with warm water, massage a little of the shampoo gently but firmly over the entire scalp. Rinse off and repeat. Rinse thoroughly and dry. Repeat at each bath until the scalp is clear and then use as necessary. Avoid contact with the eyes.     DDD

## Dentinox Infant Colic Drops

An alcohol-free suspension for the relief of wind and griping pains in infants, caused by the accumulation of ingested air. Helps to bring up wind. Can be used from birth onwards. Contains activated dimethicone (to break down wind), sucrose and parabens, a preservative.     DDD

## Dentinox Teething Gel

A sugar-free gel to relieve the pain of baby teething, containing lignocaine hydrochloride and cetylpyridinium chloride. Application can be repeated after 20 minutes if necessary.
DDD

## Dentogen Clove Oil Liquid

For the temporary relief of toothache due to a dental cavity. Prolonged use of this product should be avoided.
CUPAL

## Dentogen Ibuprofen Tablets

For the relief of toothache and the pain and swelling following minor oral surgery. Not suitable for children under 12.

Dosage: an initial dose of two tablets to be taken with water. If the dental pain continues, the initial dose may be followed by further doses of one or two tablets every four hours. Maximum dose – six tablets in 24 hours.     CUPAL

## Dequacaine

Lozenges to treat severe sore throats, containing a local anaesthetic, benzocaine, and an antibacterial agent and antifungal drug, dequalinium chloride. Not suitable for children under 12.

Dosage: adults and children over 12 – one lozenge to be sucked every two hours or as needed. No more than eight lozenges in any 24-hour period.     EVANS MEDICAL

## Dequadin

Antibacterial lozenges with dequalinium chloride (see above) for treatment of infections of the mouth and throat. Dosage for adults and children – one lozenge to be sucked slowly and repeated as necessary, or as directed by your doctor.          EVANS MEDICAL

## Derbac-M Liquid

Malathion liquid to eradicate head lice, crab lice and the scabies mite. A gentle formula ideal for use if asthma or sensitive skin is a problem. Not for infants less than six months old. For head lice – keep head upright and rub the liquid well in until the scalp and all hair is thoroughly moistened. Pay particular attention to the area around the ears and at the back of the neck. Allow hair to dry naturally. Shampoo next day with an ordinary shampoo. Use a nit comb to remove dead eggs.

INTERNATIONAL LABORATORIES

## Derbac Shampoo

Shampoo with carbaryl to eradicate head lice. Wet hair and massage into the scalp. Rinse out thoroughly. Re-apply shampoo and work into a lather. Leave on the head for at least five minutes and then rinse off with clean water. Comb out hair with a nit comb and then dry. Apply as directed at three-day intervals for a total of three applications. Not to be used on infants less than six months old.

INTERNATIONAL LABORATORIES

## Dermacort

Hydrocortisone cream for effective relief from skin irritations, dermatitis and rashes caused by plants, insect bites, jewellery, detergents and toiletries such as deodorants and soaps. Dosage: adults and children over 10 only – apply sparingly over a small area once or twice a day. Rub gently into the skin until the cream disappears. Do not use for longer than a week.

PANPHARMA

## Dermidex

Dermatological cream to soothe the irritation of itching skin and fight infection. Useful for itching, chapped hands, minor vulval and anal irritations, after-shave soreness, chafed skin, painful skin and deodorant irritation. Contains the local pain-relievers lidocaine and clorbutanol; an astringent, aluminium chlorhydroxy-allantoinate; and cetrimide, an antiseptic.

INTERNATIONAL LABORATORIES

## Dettol
Liquid antiseptic/disinfectant containing chloroxylenol for antiseptic wound cleansing and disinfection of skin lesions and abrasions, cuts, bites and insect stings. Can also be used as a germicidal agent for dandruff, spots and pimples. Should not be used in eczematous conditions. For wound cleansing and disinfection, dilute by 50 ml to one litre of water. Also available as cream and mouthwash.　　RECKITT & COLMAN

## Dijex
Indigestion tablets containing the antacids aluminium hydroxide and magnesium carbonate co-dried gel.

Dosage: adults and children over 12 – one or two tablets every two to four hours as required. Chew or swallow with a little water or milk. To relieve symptoms during the night, two tablets may be taken at bedtime. Children 5–12 years – half the above dose.　　CROOKES HEA THCARE

## Dimotane Co
A sugar-free cough medicine for dry, irritating coughs with nasal congestion. Contains pseudoephedrine hydrochloride, a decongestant; brompheniramine maleate, an antihistamine; and codeine phosphate, a cough-suppressant. May cause drowsiness. Not recommended for children under two.

Dosage, to be taken three times daily: adults, two 5 ml spoonfuls. Children 6–12 years – one and a half 5 ml spoonfuls; 4–6 years – one 5 ml spoonful; 2–4 years – half a 5 ml spoonful.　　A.H. ROBINS

## Dimotane Co Paediatric
Dimotane Co for dry, irritating coughs with nasal congestion in children. May cause drowsiness. Not recommended for children under two.

Dosage, to be taken three times a day: children 6–12 years – three 5 ml spoonfuls; 4–6 years – two 5 ml spoonfuls; 2–4 years – one 5 ml spoonful. If your child is taking other medication, or receiving medical treatment, consult your doctor before using this product.　　A.H. ROBINS

## Dimotane Expectorant
Sugar-free expectorant for chesty coughs and congestion, with guaiphenesin, an expectorant; brompheniramine maleate, an antihistamine; and pseudoephedrine hydrochloride, a decongestant. May cause drowsiness. Not

recommended for children under two.

Dosage, to be taken three times daily: adults – one or two 5 ml spoonfuls. Children 6–12 years – half to one 5 ml spoonful; 2–6 years – half a 5 ml spoonful.          A.H. ROBINS

## Dimotapp Elixir

Sugar-free nasal decongestant with the antihistamine brompheniramine maleate and decongestants phenylephrine hydrochloride and phenylpropanolamine hydrochloride. May cause drowsiness.

Dosage, to be taken three times daily: adults – one or two 5 ml spoonfuls. Children 6–12 years – one 5 ml spoonful; 2–6 years – half a 5 ml spoonful. In no instance should the interval between doses be less than four hours. If you are under the care of a doctor, are taking continual prescribed medication or you think you may be pregnant, consult your doctor before taking Dimotapp Elixir.

A.H. ROBINS

## Dimotapp Elixir Paediatric

Dimotapp Elixir for the treatment of colds, hay fever and nasal congestion in children. May cause drowsiness.

Dosage, to be taken three times daily: children 6–12 years – two 5 ml spoonfuls; 2–6 years – one 5 ml spoonful. In no instance should the interval between doses be less than four hours.          A.H. ROBINS

## Dimotapp L. A.

Tablets to help stop a runny nose caused by colds, hay fever, catarrh or nasal congestion, with the same active ingredients and safety warnings as Dimotapp Elixir, above. Not recommended for children under 12.

Dosage: one tablet night and morning.          A.H. ROBINS

## Disprin

Soluble aspirin for the relief of headache, toothache, neuralgia, period pain, rheumatic pain, lumbago, sciatica and to relieve the symptoms of colds, influenza and sore throat. Dissolve tablets in water before taking. Adults and children over 12 years: one to three tablets every four hours as needed. Do not take more than 13 tablets in 24 hours. As with other pain relievers, do not take if you have a stomach disorder. Consult your doctor before taking Disprin if you are asthmatic, allergic to aspirin or are receiving regular medical treatment.

RECKITT & COLMAN

## Disprin Extra
Tablets containing aspirin and paracetamol for the treatment of mild to moderate pain, including headache, migraine, neuralgia, toothache, sore throat, aches and pains. Also for symptomatic relief of rheumatic aches and pains, influenza, feverishness, feverish colds. Adults and children over 12: one to two tablets every four hours. Maximum six tablets in 24 hours. Not for children under 12 except on medical advice.

RECKITT & COLMAN

## Disprol
Paracetamol tablets for the treatment of mild to moderate pain, including headache, migraine, neuralgia, toothache, sore throat, period pains, aches and pains such as muscle pains and back ache. Also for symptomatic relief of rheumatic aches and pains, influenza, feverishness and feverish colds.

Dosage – adults and children over 12: one to two tablets every four hours. Maximum eight tablets in 24 hours. Children 6–12 years: half to one tablet every four hours. Maximum four tablets in 24 hours. Not to be given to children under 6 except on a doctor's advice.

RECKITT & COLMAN

## Junior Disprol Suspension
A sugar-free suspension of paracetamol in a banana-flavoured liquid for the treatment of mild to moderate pain, including headache, migraine, neuralgia, toothache, pain in teething, sore throat, aches and pains. Also for symptomatic relief of rheumatic aches and pains, influenza, feverishness and feverish colds.

Dosage: children 3–12 months: half to one 5 ml spoonful every four hours. One year to under 6 years: one to two 5 ml spoonfuls every four hours. 6–12 years: two to four 5 ml spoonfuls every four hours. No more than four doses in any 24-hour period. Dosage for children under three months at the physician's discretion.

RECKITT & COLMAN

## Doan's
Tablets containing paracetamol and sodium salicylate, a mild pain-reliever, for the relief of back pain.

Dosage: two to three tablets every four hours. Maximum 16 tablets in 24 hours.

CIBA CONSUMER

## Dr Valnet's Climarome
A natural inhalant with essential oils of lavender, niaouli, pine, mint and thyme.

Spray on a clean handkerchief or tissue and breathe in as required through the day. Alternatively, spray on to a pillow before going to sleep, or use in a bowl of hot water and inhale vapours.   CEDAR HEALTH

## Dr Valnet's Flexarome
Soothes muscular fatigue and sensitive joints. Contains ginger tincture and essential oils of origanum, common juniper, cypress, turpentine and rosemary.

LABORATOIRE COSBIONAT

## Dr Valnet's Tegarome
Natural first-aid treatment for minor abrasions, bites, burns and stings. Contains essential oils of lavender, niaouli, cypress, rosemary, sage, geranium, thyme and eucalyptus.   LABORATOIRE COSBIONAT

## Dr Valnet's Volarome
Insect-repellant with essential oils of lavender, geranium, sage, citronella, eucalyptus and mint. Apply to exposed parts of the body.

LABORATOIRE COSBIONAT

## Do-Do
Tablets for the relief of chest congestion, containing ephedrine hydrochloride, a decongestant; the stimulant caffeine; and theophylline sodium glycinate, used to treat bronchial asthma.

Dosage: one tablet every four hours with a maximum of four tablets in any 24 hours.   CIBA CONSUMER

## Do-Do Expectorant
Linctus with expectorant guaiphenesin for the relief of bronchial cough.

Dosage: adults only – two 5 ml spoonfuls four times a day.

CIBA CONSUMER

## Drapolene Cream
A cream for the prevention and treatment of nappy rash that won't block the action of one-way nappy liners or disposable nappies. Can also be used for minor burns and wounds. Contains the antiseptics benzalkonium chloride solution and cetrimide.

For nappy rash – apply evenly at every nappy change, paying particular attention to the folds of the skin. For minor burns and wounds – apply liberally to the affected area as necessary. It's important to ensure that the affected area is free from all traces of soap.   WELLCOME

## Dristan
Nasal spray for the relief of symptoms of head colds and hay fever. Contains the decongestant oxymetazoline

hydrochloride to give relief from stuffed-up nose, catarrh and nasal congestion. Also contains camphor, menthol and eucalyptus. Use only as directed. With head upright, place nozzle loosely into each nostril. Spray once or twice into each nostril, repeat every eight to ten hours as necessary. For children 6–16 years, spray lightly once into each nostril.                WHITEHALL

## Dristan Decongestant Tablets

To clear congestion and relieve pain and for the relief of colds, sinus congestion and catarrh. Contain aspirin to relieve the aches and pains associated with the common cold and flu; the decongestant phenylephrine hydrochloride; the antihistamine chlorpheniramine maleate; and the stimulant caffeine. May cause drowsiness. Not suitable for children under 12 except on medical advice.

Dosage: adults – two tablets every four hours. No more than eight tablets in 24 hours.

WHITEHALL

## Dual-Lax

Herbal laxative tablets for the relief of temporary constipation. Based on senna and cascara sagrada, herbs with a long tradition of use to relieve constipation. Available in normal strength and extra strong. Suitable for vegetarians. Gluten free. Do not use during early pregnancy or if breast-feeding.                LANES

## Dulcolax

Tablets containing the laxative bisacodyl for the relief of constipation. Also available in suppository form.

Dosage: adults and children over 10 years – two tablets at night or one 10 mg suppository in the morning. Children 6–10 years – one tablet at night or one 5 mg suppository in the morning.

WINDSOR PHARMACEUTICALS

## Duofilm

A clear paint for the treatment of plantar and mosaic warts containing the keratolytics salicylic acid and lactic acid. Warts should be soaked in hot water for five minutes. Dry with your own towel. Rub surface of warts with a pumice stone or emery board. Apply Duofilm to the warts. Allow to dry and cover with plaster if wart is large or on the foot. Continue treatment once or twice daily until the wart is completely cleared and the ridge lines of the skin have been restored.

STIEFEL

### Dusk Insect-Repellant Cream

Containing diethyltoluamide, an insect-repellant. For full protection against midges, mosquitoes and other biting insects cover all exposed areas thoroughly.    CUPAL

### Earex

Ear drops containing arachis, almond and rectified camphor oil to remove excess ear wax. To use, tilt the head to one side. Put four drops into the ear using the dropper. Gently place a piece of cotton wool into the ear and leave for about 30 minutes. Repeat night and morning for up to four days until wax is softened.    INTERNATIONAL LABORATORIES

### Emulsiderm

An emollient containing the moisturisers liquid paraffin and isopropyl myristate, with a mild antiseptic, benzalkonium chloride. Used to treat dry skin conditions such as eczema, dermatitis and psoriasis. Contains no lanolin, perfume or steroids. Can be used in the bath or as an in-shower moisturiser. Alternatively, apply directly on to the skin to treat localised dry patches. Suitable for adults and children.

DERMAL LABORATORIES

### Endekay Dental Health Gum

Chewable gum to neutralise plaque acid. Contains urea, a mild diuretic. No sugar, added colouring or preservatives. Recommended for everyone with natural teeth, both adults and children.    STAFFORD-MILLER

### Endekay Fluoride Tablets and Drops

For strengthening tooth enamel to resist decay in children. Drops for children under 2; tablets available in two strengths, for 2 to 4-year-olds and for children over 4.

Dosage – drops: serve seven drops on a spoon or mixed with food or drink. Tablets, for children 2–4 years – one tablet to be sucked or slowly dissolved in the mouth. Tablets for 4 years and over – as above.    STAFFORD-MILLER

### Eurax

Cream and lotion containing crotamiton, which relieves itching, used to treat skin irritations, except areas of dermatitis. Apply as required but only on small areas of skin in babies and infants.

CIBA CONSUMER

### Ex-Lax Pills

Laxative pills containing yellow phenolphthalein. Take with a glass of water at bedtime. Adults and children over 6 years – one pill.

INTERCARE

## Ex-Lax Tablets

Chocolate tablets with yellow phenolphthalein to relieve constipation. Take with a glass of water at bedtime. Adults one tablet. Children over 6 years – half to one tablet.

INTERCARE

## Expelix

Worm elixir with piperazine citrate to expel threadworms and roundworms from the gastro-intestinal tract. For threadworms, take daily for seven days. It may be necessary to repeat the dosage after seven days for a further seven days.

Dosage: adults and children over 12 – three 5 ml spoonfuls. Children 7–12 years – two 5 ml spoonfuls; 4–6 years – one and a half 5 ml spoonfuls; 2–3 years – one 5 ml spoonful; under one year – on medical advice only.

To expel roundworms – dosage to be taken as single dose and then repeated after 14 days. Adults and children over 12 – six 5 ml spoonfuls. Children 9–12 years – five 5 ml spoonfuls; 6–8 years four 5 ml spoonfuls; 4–5 years – three 5 ml spoonfuls; 1–3 years – two 5 ml spoonfuls;

under one year – on medical advice only.

CUPAL

## Exterol Ear Drops

A solution containing urea hydrogen peroxide to soften and effervesce within the ear wax – helping to break down its structure and expel it naturally. This special action may be heard as a slight bubbling in the ear. Squeeze five to ten drops into the ear. Retain in the ear for a few minutes by keeping the head tilted. Repeat once or twice a day for at least three or four days.

DERMAL LABORATORIES

## Famel Catarrh and Throat Pastilles

Pastilles containing creosote, a disinfectant, and soothing menthol, for the relief of sore, infected throats, catarrh and coughs. Suck one pastille as required.

OPTREX (CROOKES HEALTHCARE)

## Famel Expectorant

Linctus with the expectorant guaiphenesin and liquid glucose for the relief of tight, chesty coughs.

Dosage: adults and children over 12 – four 5 ml spoonfuls. Children 5–12 years – two 5 ml spoonfuls; 1–5 years – one 5 ml spoonful. Take the dose every four hours up to four times daily.

OPTREX (CROOKES HEALTHCARE)

### Famel Honey and Lemon Cough Pastilles

Pastilles to soothe coughs and sore throats, containing the expectorant guaiphenesin. Not recommended for children under five.

Dosage: adults and children over 10 – one every hour as required. Children 5–10 years – one every two hours.

OPTREX (CROOKES HEALTHCARE)

### Famel Linctus

For the relief of dry, tickly coughs. Containing pholcodine, a cough-suppressant, and papaverine hydrochloride, used to treat spasm of smooth muscle.

Dosage: adults and children over 12 – two 5 ml spoonfuls; children 5–12 years – one 5 ml spoonful. Not suitable for children under five, except on medical advice.

OPTREX (CROOKES HEALTHCARE)

### Famel Original

Syrup for the symptomatic relief of dry, troublesome coughs. Contains creosote, a disinfectant often used in small doses in cough mixtures, and codeine phosphate, a cough-suppressant. May cause drowsiness.

Dosage: adults and children over 12 – two to three 5 ml spoonfuls; in acute cases, three to four 5 ml spoonfuls.

Not suitable for children under 12.

OPTREX (CROOKES HEALTHCARE)

### Feminax

Painkillers specially formulated to ease period pain and associated stomach cramps, back ache and headache. Contain paracetamol; codeine phosphate, a mild pain-reliever; caffeine, a stimulant; and hyoscine hydrobromide, used to relieve spasm in abdominal and pelvic muscles. May cause drowsiness. Not recommended for children under 12. Not to be taken by persons suffering from glaucoma.

Dosage: adults and girls over 12 – up to two tablets every four hours. No more than six tablets in 24 hours.

NICHOLAS

### Fennings Adult Powders

Paracetamol and caffeine powders for the treatment of headaches, migraine, period pains and for the relief of symptoms of flu and feverish colds.

Dosage: adults and children over 12 only – one or two powders in water every four hours as needed. Do not repeat less than three hours after each dose or take more than eight doses in any 24-hour period.   FENNINGS

## Fennings Children's Cooling Powders

Paracetamol powders for the treatment of pain arising from teething, headache, aches, pains and the symptomatic relief of feverish colds, flu and mild feverish conditions.

Dosage, to a maximum of four doses daily: babies 3 months to 1 year – one powder; children 1 year to under 6 years – two powders. The powder may be given in a little milk or jam.   FENNINGS

## Fennings Gripe Mixture

Contains the antacid sodium bicarbonate, ginger tincture, peppermint oil, dill oil and caraway oil to relieve wind and griping pains and tummy upsets.

Dosage: babies 1–6 months – one 5 ml spoonful; 6 months to 2 years – two 5 ml spoonfuls. Children over 2 years – two to three 5 ml spoonfuls.   FENNINGS

## Fennings Lemon-Flavoured Mixture

Sodium salicylate mixture (a mild pain-reliever) for the symptomatic relief of flu, feverishness, feverish colds, rheumatic pain, sprains,

strains, lumbago, fibrositis and muscular pains.

One dose to be taken every four hours with an equal quantity of water. Adults – four 5 ml spoonfuls. No more than four doses in 24 hours. Not recommended for children. Do not take if you have a stomach ulcer.   FENNINGS

## Fenox Nasal Drops

To relieve nasal congestion due to head colds, catarrh, blocked sinuses and hay fever. Contains phenylephrine hydrochloride, a decongestant. Use morning and night and every four hours if necessary. Don't use drops for longer than seven days without medical advice.

CROOKES HEALTHCARE

## Fiery Jack Rubbing Ointment

Rub containing capsicum and one of the hottest on the market for back ache, muscular aches and pains, lumbago, and stiff joints. To be applied once or twice daily only, and only to a limited area of skin overlying the painful area. Not to be used by people with delicate or sensitive skin. Never apply to diseased or broken skin. Care should also be taken to avoid sensitive parts of the body and to wash the hands thoroughly after use. Avoid contact with clothing as ointment may stain.                 J. PICKLES & SONS

### Flurex

Decongestant inhalant capsules for the relief of nasal congestion in head colds, catarrh, flu and hay fever for adults, children and babies. Contains camphor, menthol, turpentine oil and eucalyptus oil. Empty one capsule into hot water and inhale vapour freely. For young children, empty a capsule on to a handkerchief and tie it down securely in the vicinity.   CUPAL

### Flurex Bedtime Medicine

For the night-time symptomatic relief of colds and flu. Liquid contains paracetamol, diphenhydramine hydrochloride, an antihistamine, and pseudo-ephedrine hydrochloride, a decongestant. May cause drowsiness. Asthmatics should consult their doctor before using this product. Do not use during pregnancy.

Dosage: adults and children over 12 only – take 20 ml at bedtime (use measure supplied). Do not exceed the stated dose.   CUPAL

### Flurex Capsules

Capsules containing paracetamol and phenylephrine hydrochloride to clear a stuffy nose for the short-term symptomatic relief of colds and flu. Not recommended for children under 6. Not to be taken during pregnancy or while breast-feeding.

Dosage: adults and children over 12 – two capsules to be taken four-hourly. Not more than 12 capsules a day. Children 6–12 years – one capsule to be taken four-hourly. Not more than six capsules a day.   CUPAL

### Flurex Hot Lemon Syrup

Hot lemon drink containing codeine phosphate, a cough-suppressant; ephedrine hydrochloride, a decongestant; and diphenhydramine hydrochloride, an antihistamine. For the symptomatic relief of colds, flu and associated dry cough. Not recommended for children under 12. May cause drowsiness. Not to be used during pregnancy.

Dosage: two 5 ml spoonfuls three or four times a day at three-hourly intervals. Dilute with half a cup of hot water.   CUPAL

## Flurex Tablets

Contain paracetamol, the stimulant caffeine and phenylephrine hydrochloride to clear a stuffy nose. Used for the short-term symptomatic relief of colds, flu and catarrh. Not to be taken during pregnancy or when breast-feeding. Not for children under six.

Dosage: adults and children over 12 – one or two tablets to be taken four-hourly as needed. For light infections the dose may be reduced to one tablet every three hours. No more than eight tablets a day. Children 6–12 years – one tablet four-hourly if required. No more than four tablets per day.          CUPAL

## Franolyn Expect.

For tight, chesty coughs with congestion. Contains the expectorant guaiphenesin; theophylline to ease congested airways; and ephedrine, a decongestant.

Dosage: adults – two 5 ml spoonfuls. Children 7–12 years – one 5 ml spoonful. Repeat up to four times a day if necessary. Children under 7 – on medical advice only. Take with or after food. May occasionally interfere with sleep, in which case the evening dose should be reduced. Asthmatics should consult their doctor before using this product.

JANSSEN PHARMACEUTICAL

## Franolyn Sed.

Syrup for the relief of dry, irritating coughs, containing dextromethorphan hydrobromide, a cough-suppressant.

Dosage: adults – two 5 ml spoonfuls. Children 7–12 years, one 5 ml spoonful. Children under seven – on medical advice only.

JANSSEN PHARMACY DIVISION

## Freezone Liquid

A liquid corn-remover containing salicylic acid. Soak the affected foot in warm water for 15 minutes. Dry thoroughly, then rub the corn very gently with a pumice stone to remove any dead skin. Apply Freezone a drop at a time until the corn is covered. Cover with a waterproof plaster. Repeat daily, renewing the plaster each time until the corn can be lifted out.          WHITEHALL

## Full Marks Shampoo

Shampoo containing phenothrin insecticide for the treatment of head lice. Wet hair thoroughly with warm water, apply sufficient shampoo to work up a rich lather and leave for at least five minutes. Rinse thoroughly with clean, warm water. Repeat. While hair is still wet, comb out tangles with an ordinary comb. Use a nit comb to remove dead lice and eggs.                      NAPP

### Gastrils Antacid Pastilles

Pastilles containing aluminium hydroxide and magnesium carbonate co-dried gel for the relief of indigestion, heartburn, flatulence and dyspepsia. Not suitable for children under 12. Suck or chew two pastilles as needed. Repeat whenever discomfort is felt, but do not take more than 12 pastilles in any 12-hour period.           ERNEST JACKSON

### Gaviscon

Liquid for the relief of heartburn and indigestion due to gastric reflux. Contains the antacids sodium alginate, sodium bicarbonate and calcium carbonate. Adults and children over 12: two to four 5 ml spoonfuls after meals and at bedtime, or as directed. This may be followed by a drink of water if desired. If your doctor has advised a low salt diet, please note that each 10 ml contains 141 mg of sodium. Also available in tablet form.       RECKITT & COLMAN

### Gee's Linctus

Pastilles to relieve stubborn coughs. Not suitable for children under 12. Contain concentrated camphorated opium tincture (to suppress an unnecessary cough), squill liquid extract (an expectorant), cinnamic acid and benzoic acid (antiseptics), glacial acetic acid (an expectorant) and honey. Suck two pastilles every four hours and at bedtime.
                      ERNEST JACKSON

### Gelusil

Antacid tablets for the relief of hyperacidity, indigestion and heartburn whether occurring alone or in association with a peptic ulcer. Contain magnesium trisilicate and dried aluminium hydroxide.

Dosage: adults – one or two tablets to be chewed or sucked after meals or whenever symptoms arise. Children 6–12 years – half or one tablet. Gelusil tablets contain 561 mg sugar per tablet, so patients suffering from diabetes should seek their doctor's advice first if this is the antacid they prefer to take.          WARNER LAMBERT

### Genisol

Lotion containing sodium sulphosuccinated undecylenic mono-alkyloamide (an antifungal agent) and purified coal tar fractions to treat dandruff. Wet hair thoroughly and use approximately 10 ml of Genisol as a shampoo. Work well into the scalp with fingers, rinse and repeat. Keep away from eyes. FISONS

## Gluco-lyte

Oral rehydration treatment containing essential mineral salts – sodium chloride, potassium chloride, sodium bicarbonate and glucose monohydrate – for the treatment of diarrhoea and fluid loss in infants, children and adults. Pour contents into a glass and add 200 ml of fresh drinking water. For infants and where drinking water isn't available, use freshly boiled and cooled water. Stir until powder has completely dissolved.

Dosage: adults and children over 12 – use one or two reconstituted sachets after each loose bowel movement. Children 1–12 years – use one reconstituted sachet after each loose bowel movement. Infants – substitute equivalent volumes of reconstituted solution in place of feeds, or give the appropriate volume before breast-feeding. Artificial or cow's milk feeds should be re-introduced

gradually when diarrhoea has lessened. CUPAL

## Glutarol

Wart treatment containing the disinfectant glutaraldehyde. Gently rub the surface of the wart with a pumice stone or emery board, or pare down any hard skin. Apply a few drops of paint to the wart. Repeat twice daily. There is no need to use a sticking plaster.
DERMAL LABORATORIES

## Gonne Balm

A warming balm of menthol, camphor and oils of cajuput, eucalyptus, turpentine and methyl salicylate – a counter-irritant. Particularly useful as a pre-sports rub. Apply with gentle massage two or three times daily and also at night if necessary. For maximum effect have a hot bath first. This opens the pores and ensures deeper penetration. LANES

## HC45 Hydrocortisone Cream

For treatment of contact dermatitis caused by allergies or irritants and of skin reactions to insect bites. Contains hydrocortisone acetate which reduces inflammation and calms irritated skin. Use sparingly on a small area, once or twice a day for a maximum of seven days. If the condition doesn't improve, consult your doctor. Do not use on the eyes, face, anal or genital areas, or on broken or infected skin such as that caused by impetigo, cold sores, acne or athlete's foot. Do not use during pregnancy or for children under 10 without medical advice.                CROOKES HEALTHCARE

## Hedex and Hedex Extra

Easy-to-swallow paracetamol caplets designed for relief from headaches, but effective for treatment of back ache, rheumatic and muscle pains, period pain and toothache. Also relieves fever, aches and pains associated with colds and flu. Hedex Extra contains the stimulant caffeine, so avoid drinking too much tea or coffee while taking these tablets.

Hedex is not suitable for children under six. Dosage: adults – two caplets up to four times daily. No more than eight in 24 hours. Children 6–12 years – half or one caplet up to four times daily. No more than four in 24 hours. Do not repeat more frequently than every four hours. Take with a tumblerful of water.

Hedex Extra: adults only –

two caplets up to four times daily. No more frequently than every four hours, and no more than eight caplets in 24 hours.

Hedex is also available in soluble form – each sachet contains a complete adult dose of paracetamol. Add the contents to a tumblerful of water and stir. Drink when effervescence subsides. Take one sachet up to four times daily – no more than four sachets in 24 hours and no more frequently than every four hours.                STERLING HEALTH

## Heemex

A soothing, healing ointment containing hamamelis (witch-hazel), compound tinct benzoine and zinc oxide (protective agents). For the symptomatic relief of discomfort, itching and irritation due to internal and external piles. Adults and the elderly should apply Heemex freely night and morning and after every bowel movement.
                LANES

## Hemocane Suppositories

Suppositories with five ingredients for all-round relief from symptoms of painful internal piles. Contains a local anaesthetic, lignocaine hydrochloride; soothing protective agents zinc oxide and bismuth oxide to help heal raw, tender tissues; benzoic acid, an antiseptic; and cinnamic acid, an antibacterial and antifungal agent. Use one suppository morning and night, and after bowel movements.            INTERCARE

## Herbal Laboratories' Herbal Feverfew 125

Tablets containing organically grown feverfew leaf powder which many people have found helpful in the treatment of migraine.            CEDAR HEALTH

## Herbelix Specific

A traditional remedy to help relieve catarrh, mucous congestion, rhinitis, head colds and hay fever. The active ingredients are lobelia ethereal tinct, tolu solution and sodium bicarbonate. Suitable for vegans and vegetarians. Gluten free.

Dosage: adults – one 5 ml spoonful taken in a little water at bedtime. Children 7–14 years – half a 5 ml spoonful.
                     LANES

## Hismanal

Tablets containing the antihistamine astemizole to relieve hay fever without causing drowsiness. Dosage: adults and children over 12 – one tablet once a day on an empty stomach, preferably in the morning. Do not take Hismanal if you are or may be pregnant, or are breast-feeding. Since people vary in their response to medications, it may take two to three days to attain maximum effect. For best results, take Hismanal continuously every day for as long as the hay-fever season lasts.          JANSSEN PHARMACEUTICAL

## Hofels Original and One-A-Day Garlic Pearls

A traditional herbal remedy for the relief of catarrh, symptoms of rhinitis and other symptoms of common colds and coughs. Dosage – Original: adults three capsules daily, either one before each meal or three before bed. Children 7–12 years – two capsules daily. Dosage: One-A-Day – one capsule a day, preferably with a meal.

Garlic tablets are also available with parsley – take one tablet three times a day before meals.     HOFELS PURE FOODS

## Hypercal Cream

A topical herbal remedy traditionally used in the symptomatic treatment of cuts and sores. Combines the healing qualities of calendula (marigold) with the pain-relieving properties of hypericum (St John's Wort).

Apply to more than cover the affected area. Cover with plain lint and bandage if necessary.                    NELSONS

## Ibuleve

A clear, fragrance-free gel containing the pain-reliever ibuprofen. Designed to be rapidly absorbed into the skin for effective relief at the point of pain and inflammation associated with conditions such as back ache, rheumatic and muscular pain, sprains, strains and neuralgia.

Lightly apply a thin layer of the gel over the affected area. Massage gently until absorbed. Repeat as needed up to three times daily. If symptoms persist for more than a few weeks consult your doctor. Not recommended for children under 14. Patients with a history of kidney problems should seek medical advice before using Ibuleve. Keep away from broken skin, lips and eyes. Not to be used during pregnancy or while breast-feeding.                    DDD

## Imodium

Tablets containing loperamide hydrochloride, which slows down gut wall muscles to treat diarrhoea. Not recommended for children under 12.

Dosage: two capsules initially, followed by one capsule after each further loose bowel movement up to a maximum of eight a day.

JANSSEN PHARMACEUTICAL

## Indigestion Lozenges

Antacid lozenges containing calcium carbonate, heavy magnesium carbonate and bismuth carbonate for the relief of indigestion. Take one or two lozenges after each meal.                    ERNEST JACKSON

## Inoven

Ibuprofen caplets to relieve pain, reduce inflammation and lower temperature. Effective in the relief of headaches, symptoms of colds and flu, muscular pain, rheumatic pain, back ache, neuralgia, migraine, period pain and dental pain.

Dosage: adults and children over 12 – initial dose two caplets with water, followed by one or two caplets every four hours if necessary. No more than six caplets in 24 hours. Not suitable for children under 12.

JANSSEN PHARMACEUTICAL

## Kalms Tablets

A traditional herbal remedy containing extracts of valerian, hops and gentian to help relieve periods of anxiety, stresses and strains and allow restful sleep. No known evidence of habit-forming effects. Not suitable for children.

Dosage: two tablets three times a day after meals. Do not take during pregnancy or while breast-feeding. Seek medical advice if you're taking other medications or if the condition worsens.          LANES

## Karvol Decongestant Capsules

A combination of natural oils, including pine, cinammon and menthol, to help clear nasal congestion. Suitable for children and adults. Empty one capsule into hot water and inhale vapour freely. For young children, empty a capsule on to a handkerchief and tie it down securely in the vicinity.          CROOKES HEALTHCARE

## Kwells and Junior Kwells

Melt-in-the-mouth anti-travel sickness tablets containing hyoscine hydrobromide to control motion sickness and nausea caused by disturbances of the inner ear. May cause drowsiness. Can be taken up to 30 minutes before start of journey, or at the onset of nausea. Not to be taken by persons suffering from glaucoma. Children should not be left unattended.

Dosage: Kwells – adults, one tablet every six hours if needed. No more than three in 24 hours. Children over 10 – half to one tablet, not more than one and a half to three in 24 hours; 4–10 years – half a tablet, not more than one and a half in 24 hours. Children under 4 – only on medical advice. It is dangerous to exceed the stated dose.

Junior Kwells: children 7–12 years – one to two tablets, not more than three to six in 24 hours; 3–7 years – half to one tablet, not more than one and a half to three in 24 hours. Children under 3 – only on medical advice.          NICHOLAS

## Lacto-Calamine

Soothing calamine lotion with protective zinc oxide, cooling hamamelis water and phenol, for relieving discomfort caused by skin irritations, sunburn, insect bites and stings. Apply as needed.

KIRBY-WARRICK

## Lanacane

Soothing cream containing the local anaesthetic benzocaine, resorcinol to stop itching and chlorothymol, an antiseptic, for the relief of itching and pain of everyday scrapes and cuts, heat rash, nettle rash, itchy, dry skin, sore 'detergent hands', eczema, rectal or vaginal itching. Apply cream to affected area as needed three or four times daily. Not for prolonged use.

COMBE INTERNATIONAL

## Lanacort Creme and Ointment

Hydrocortisone creme and ointment to calm the body's reactions to skin disturbances and aid healing. For relief from rashes, redness, itching, skin irritations, inflammation and scaling caused by insect bites, stings and allergic reactions to soaps, jewellery, toiletries and detergents. Maximum strength available without prescription. Use sparingly over a small area once or twice daily for a maximum period of one week. Do not use during pregnancy or for children under 10 without medical advice. Do not use on the eyes, face, ano-genital region, broken or infected skin including that caused by cold sores, acne and athlete's foot.   COMBE INTERNATIONAL

## Lana-sting Creme

For relief from the itch and irritation of insect bites, stings and nettle rash. Contains the gentle anaesthetic lignocaine and the antiseptic benzyl alcohol. Apply liberally to the affected area. Repeat as needed three to four times daily. Do not use for more than five days. Not suitable for children under one year of age. Do not get Lana-sting into eyes, mouth, nose, rectum or vagina. Not for use on deep puncture wounds or serious burns.   COMBE INTERNATIONAL

## Lana-sting Spray

Instant spray relief from the itch of sunburn, insect bites, stings and nettle rash, with the local anaesthetic benzocaine and the antiseptic benzethonium chloride. Spray liberally on the affected area. Repeat as needed three or four times daily. Not for prolonged use. Not suitable for children under one year of age. Do not spray into eyes, mouth, nose, rectum or vagina. Not for use on deep puncture wounds or serious burns.   COMBE INTERNATIONAL

## Lanes Balto Foot Balm

A natural blend of camphor, menthol, oils of pine and bladderwrack, protective zinc oxide and precipitated sulphur, a mild antiseptic. To soften hard, cracked skin, help curb excessive perspiration and cool tired, aching feet. Rub ointment into affected area night and morning.   LANES

## Lanes Charcoal Tablets

Said to absorb excess gas in the intestinal tract, relieving flatulence and heartburn and also thought to be helpful in treating dyspepsia and occasional diarrhoea.   LANES

## Lasonil

An ointment for bruises, sprains, piles and soft-tissue injuries. Contains heparinoid, an anti-inflammatory agent, and hyaluronidase, an enzyme which makes tissue more permeable. Unless otherwise directed, apply thickly to the affected area two to three times daily. If symptoms persist, consult your doctor. For external use only.   BAYER

## Laxoberal

A laxative containing sodium picosulphate, which is broken down by bacteria in the large intestine to form soft stools usually 10–14 hours after administration.

Dosage: adults – 5–15 ml at night. Children 5–10 years – 2.5–5 ml at night; children 0–5 years – 2.5 ml at night.

WINDSOR PHARMACEUTICALS

## Lemsip

Powder containing paracetamol, phenylephrine hydrochloride – to constrict blood vessels and so ease congestion, ascorbic acid and sodium citrate (used as an expectorant) with real lemon for the relief of the symptoms of colds and influenza such as aches and pains and nasal congestion, and for the lowering of temperature. Also available in blackcurrant flavour.

Dosage – adults and children over 12: one sachet dissolved by stirring in hot water. The dose may be repeated after four hours. No more than six doses should be taken in 24 hours. Not for children under 12 except on medical advice.   RECKITT & COLMAN

## Junior Lemsip

Powder containing paracetamol, phenylephrine hydrochloride – which constricts blood vessels to ease congestion, the expectorant sodium citrate and ascorbic acid for the relief of the symptoms of colds and influenza in children, including the relief of aches and pains, nasal congestion and lowering of temperature. Children 6–12 years: two sachets dissolved in a beakerful of hot (not boiling) water every four hours. Maximum eight sachets in 24 hours. Children 3 years to under 6 years: one sachet dissolved in half a beakerful of hot (not boiling) water every four hours. Maximum four sachets in 24 hours. Not to be given to children under three except on a doctor's advice.

RECKITT & COLMAN

## Lemsip Cold Relief Capsules

Capsules for the treatment of the symptoms of colds and influenza, containing paracetamol, the stimulant caffeine and phenylephrine hydrochloride, which constricts blood vessels to ease congestion. Adults and children over 12: one to two capsules every three to four hours. Do not exceed eight capsules in 24 hours. Not to be given to children under 12 without medical advice.

RECKITT & COLMAN

## Lemsip Expectorant

Raspberry-flavoured expectorant containing diphenhydramine hydrochloride (an antihistamine), ammonium chloride and sodium citrate (expectorants) to relieve chesty coughs and congestive symptoms such as phlegm and catarrh. Adults and children over 12: one or two 5 ml spoonfuls. Children 6–12: one 5 ml spoonful. The doses may be repeated at three to four-hourly intervals. Not recommended for children under six years. May cause drowsiness. Not recommended for use in pregnancy.

RECKITT & COLMAN

## Lemsip Linctus

Honey and lemon-flavoured cough linctus containing ipecacuanha liquid extract (an expectorant), honey, lemon oil, glycerol (a demulcent), and citric acid for the relief of dry, tickly coughs and to soothe sore, irritated throats. Adults and children over 12: three 5 ml spoonfuls. Children 6–12: two 5 ml spoonfuls. Children 2–6: one 5 ml spoonful. The dose may be repeated at two to three-hourly intervals. Not to be used for children under two years.

RECKITT & COLMAN

## Lenium

Dandruff treatment cream shampoo containing selenium sulphide. Use shampoo twice weekly for two weeks, once a week for a further two weeks and then every three to six weeks as required to maintain control. Use as normal shampoo, but leave second lather on scalp for five minutes. Lenium should not be used within 48 hours of perming or dyeing hair.

JANSSEN PHARMACEUTICAL

## Librofem
Tablets containing ibuprofen specifically for the relief of period pain. Take two tablets every four hours with a maximum of six tablets in 24 hours.                          CIBA

## Listerine Antiseptic
A solution for oral hygiene, bad breath and for relief of sore throats. Can also be used as an antiseptic for minor cuts, bites, stings and wounds. Contains the antiseptics benzoic acid, thymol, eucalyptol, with menthol, methyl salicylate and ethanol. For adults and children. Rinse the mouth, teeth and gums vigorously night and morning with half a mouthful of Listerine. Then tilt the head back and gargle for 30 seconds. Don't swallow.
                                WARNER LAMBERT

## Listermint
An oral antiseptic, mouthwash and breath-freshener containing cetylpyridinium chloride, an antiseptic, and zinc chloride, an astringent which 'tightens up' the gum membranes and reduces inflammation. Suitable for adults and children. Rinse the mouth or gargle with half a capful of Listermint every morning. Do not swallow. Do not dilute.
                                WARNER LAMBERT

## Lustys Garlic Perles
Herbal remedy containing essential oil of garlic, available in two potencies and traditionally used to treat the symptoms of the common cold and coughs. Can also be used for temporary relief of the symptoms of rhinitis and catarrh. The higher potency is not recommended for children under 12.

Dosage: adults – one capsule before each meal or up to three at bedtime with a little water. Children 5 to 12 – one capsule of the lower potency twice daily.
                        LUSTYS NATURAL PRODUCTS

## Lustys Herbalene
A powdered blend of dried herbs and seeds including senna leaf, buckthorn, elder leaf and fennel to help relieve temporary or occasional constipation.

Dosage: adults – half to one 5 ml spoonful placed on the tongue and washed down with a little warm water first thing in the morning and last thing at night. Children 7–14 years – half the above dose. Alternatively, Herbalene may be brewed by adding half to one 5 ml spoonful to half a cup of boiling water. Cool and strain before drinking.
                        LUSTYS NATURAL PRODUCTS

## Lyclear

A creme rinse for the treatment of head lice and their eggs. Contains permethrin, an insecticide. Used as directed a ten-minute application of the rinse will kill head lice and their eggs. As with all medicines, if you're pregnant or currently taking any other medicine, consult your doctor or pharmacist before using this product.

WELLCOME

## Lypsyl

Moisturiser for chapped lips available in original flavour, lemon and mint as well as a night-time gel in a tube. Apply as required.          CIBA

## Massage Balm

A remedy with extracts from arnica flowers, birch leaves, lavender – lavandin oil, and rosemary oil, for the relief of stiffness, fibrositis, muscular and rheumatic pain. Also for the symptomatic relief of bruising, sciatica, lumbago and cramp. Should ideally be used after a warm bath or shower, while the skin is still damp.

WELEDA

## Medicaid

Antiseptic cream containing cetrimide for sun- and wind-burned skin, sore, chapped hands, chafing in the intimate areas beneath the breasts and in the crotch, nappy rash, minor burns, cuts and grazes – whenever skin is too sore to touch. Apply liberally to the affected area. Repeat as necessary. For first aid, wash area gently and pat dry before application. For nappy rash, apply after nappy changing, paying particular attention to tiny folds and creases where irritation often begins. Give an extra application at night for protection during the baby's longest sleep period.

NEWTON CHEMICAL

## Medicinal Charcoal Biscuits and Tablets by J.L. Bragg

Contain pure vegetable charcoal for the relief of indigestion, wind and heartburn. Also relieve halitosis. Take four or more biscuits during or after meals. Tablets – take two or more after meals.          J.L. BRAGG

## Medised

Soothing blackcurrant-flavoured suspension giving pain relief for children from 3 months to 12 years old. Contains paracetamol and a mild antihistamine, promethazine hydrochloride. Reduces temperature and relieves painful or feverish conditions such as toothache, headache, sore throat, colds and flu. May cause drowsiness.

Dosage: children 6–12 years – four 5 ml spoonfuls; 1–6 years – two 5 ml spoonfuls. Babies 3 months to 1 year – one 5 ml spoonful. Under three months – on doctor's advice only. The dose should not be repeated more frequently than every four hours, and no more than four doses should be given in any 24-hour period. The suspension can be mixed with a little water or fruit juice if preferred.          PANPHARMA

## Meggozones
Pastilles containing menthol, benzoin and liquorice to soothe soreness in the throat, relieve coughs and reduce catarrh. Adults – allow one pastille to dissolve slowly in the mouth as needed. Maximum daily dosage – 15 pastilles. If the mouth becomes sensitive, irritated or sore, discontinue use.

SCHERING-PLOUGH CONSUMER HEALTH

## Meltus Adult Dry Cough Elixir
Sugar- and colour-free elixir containing dextromethorphan hydrobromide, a cough-suppressant and pseudo-ephedrine hydrochloride, a decongestant. May cause drowsiness. Asthmatics should consult their doctor before using this product.

Dosage: adults and children over 12 only – one 5 ml spoonful to be taken four times a day.          CUPAL

## Meltus Adult Expectorant and Junior
Linctus containing the expectorant guaiphenesin and cetylpyridinium chloride, an antiseptic, as well as sucrose and honey, for the symptomatic relief of coughs and catarrh in influenza, colds and mild throat infections. Not suitable for children under 12.

Dosage: one or two 5 ml spoonfuls swallowed slowly every three or four hours. Junior version – for children over two years of age. Dosage, to be taken three or four times daily: children over 6 – two 5 ml spoonfuls; 2–6 years – one 5 ml spoonful.
CUPAL

## Meltus Baby Cough Linctus
Sugar- and colour-free blackcurrant-flavoured linctus containing dilute acetic acid, an expectorant, for the symptomatic relief of irritating and distressing coughs often accompanying

colds, especially for babies over three months old and young children.

Dosage, to be given slowly: children over $2\frac{1}{2}$ years – two 5 ml spoonfuls; $1$–$2\frac{1}{2}$ years – one 5 ml spoonful. Babies 3 months to 1 year – half a 5 ml spoonful. Repeat as needed every two or three hours.

CUPAL

## Menthol and Wintergreen Heat Rub

Counter-irritant heat rub containing methyl salicylate, eucalyptus oil, camphor, menthol and mustard oil, to ease muscular pain and stiffness caused by rheumatic conditions including fibrositis and lumbago. Also effective for sprains and bruises. Apply two or three times daily over the affected muscles and joints. Massage gently but firmly.

CUPAL

## Mentholatum Vapour Rub

Blended from natural menthol and eucalyptus with extracts of pine. Also contains methyl salicylate. The vapour from these ingredients clears congestion, eases breathing and relieves soreness. Can also be used to relieve itching, insect bites and stings, nettle rash or dry skin. A nasal inhaler is also available.

MENTHOLATUM

## Merocaine

Lozenges containing an antiseptic – cetylpyridinium chloride, and a local anaesthetic – benzocaine, to relieve pain and discomfort from severe sore throat due to tonsillitis and pharyngitis. Also helpful in easing pain from gum infections. Suitable for adults and children over 12. Allow to dissolve slowly in the mouth. Take one every two hours as needed. Do not exceed eight lozenges in 24 hours. If symptoms persist or are severe, or are accompanied by fever, headache, nausea and vomiting, consult your doctor.

MERRELL DOW

## Merocets

Sore throat lozenges to soothe irritated and inflamed tissues. Contain cetylpyridinium chloride, an antibacterial agent. Suitable for adults and children over six. Dissolve slowly in the mouth. One lozenge every three hours.

MERRELL DOW

## Merothol

Lozenges to relieve sore throats due to colds and to relieve nasal congestion. Contain the antibacterial agent cetylpyridinium chloride and soothing menthol and eucalyptus oil. Suitable for adults and children over three.

Dissolve slowly in the mouth. One every three hours or as often as needed.    MERRELL DOW

## Metamucil

A natural laxative containing ispaghula husk. Adults and children over 12 should take one rounded 5 ml spoonful. Children 6–12, a quarter to one level 5 ml spoonful. Usually taken one to three times a day depending on need and response. Continued use for two to three days may be needed for most benefit. Add dosage to 150 ml cool water, milk, fruit juice or other liquid. Adequate fluid intake should be maintained. Not to be taken in cases of intestinal obstruction, faecal impaction or a previously discovered hypersensitivity to ispaghula – when it causes unpleasant diarrhoea, for example.    SEARLE CONSUMER PRODUCTS

## Migraclear

Soluble tablets containing aspirin to relieve migraine pain and cyclizine hydrochloride, an antihistamine and anti-emetic, to help prevent vomiting and reduce nausea. Tablets must be dissolved in water. May cause drowsiness. Don't take if you have a stomach ulcer, nor during pregnancy without consulting your doctor.

Dosage: two tablets at the first signs of a migraine attack. May be repeated every four hours as needed. No more than eight tablets in 24 hours. Not suitable for children under 12.    NICHOLAS

## Migraleve

Tablets to relieve migraine headache, nausea and vomiting. Not suitable for children under 10. May cause drowsiness. Pack contains eight pink and four yellow tablets. Pink tablets contain the pain-relievers paracetamol and codeine phosphate and the antihistamine buclizine hydrochloride.

Adults should take two pink tablets at the first sign of a migraine attack. If further treatment is needed, take two yellow tablets every four hours. Maximum dose – two pink and not more than six yellow tablets in 24 hours.

Children 10–14 years – take one pink tablet initially. If necessary, follow with one yellow tablet every four hours. Maximum dose – one pink and not more than three yellow tablets in 24 hours.

Yellow tablets do not contain buclizine hydrochloride.

CHARWELL PHARMACEUTICALS

## Milk of Magnesia

A stomach-upset remedy for all the family. Contains magnesium hydroxide for the relief of indigestion, over-acidity, heartburn and flatulence. Can also be used as a laxative.

Dosage: adults one to two 5 ml spoonfuls. Children 3–12 years, one 5 ml spoonful. As a laxative – adults, two to three 15 ml spoonfuls at bedtime. Repeat nightly, reducing dose each night until constipation is relieved. Children 1–12 years, one to two 5 ml spoonfuls at bedtime. Under 1 year – only as recommended by your doctor. Can be taken in milk or water if desired.

Also available in tablet form. STERLING HEALTH

## Mil-Par

A laxative emulsion containing magnesium hydroxide and liquid paraffin. Not recommended for children under 3.

Dosage: adults one to two 15 ml spoonfuls before breakfast or at bedtime. Children over 7 – half to one 15 ml spoonful at bedtime; 3–7 years – one to two 5 ml spoonfuls at bedtime. Can be mixed with half a glass of milk or water if desired.

STERLING HEALTH

## Morhulin Cod-Liver Oil Ointment

Contains cod-liver oil and zinc oxide to provide a barrier to protect baby's skin from contact exposure to moisture. Use at every nappy change.

NAPP

## Moorland

Tablets for the relief of indigestion, heartburn and flatulence. Contain the antacids bismuth aluminate, magnesium trisilicate, dried aluminium hydroxide gel, heavy magnesium carbonate, light kaolin and calcium carbonate.

Dosage: two tablets dissolved slowly in the mouth after each meal and last thing at night, or when required.

CROOKES HEALTHCARE

## Morsep Nappy-Rash Cream

Nappy-rash cream containing sunflower oil and cod-liver oil as a barrier to protect a baby's skin from constant exposure to moisture, combined with lanolin to protect and soothe, and an antibacterial agent, cetrimide, to help fight infection. Use at every nappy change. NAPP

## Mrs Cullen's Powders

Contain aspirin and caffeine for the relief of headaches, colds, flu, neuralgia, rheumatic and period pains. Not suitable for children under 12. Take a powder immediately when colds and flu symptoms are experienced. Repeat every four hours. For other pain, take one powder and repeat every three or four hours as necessary. Mix powder in a little water or fruit drink.

CULLEN AND DAVISON

## Mucron

Tablets for the relief of nasal congestion, containing phenylpropanolamine hydrochloride, which constricts blood vessels to ease congestion, and paracetamol. Take one tablet two to four times a day with a maximum of four tablets in 24 hours.

CIBA

## Mucron Junior Syrup

Syrup for the relief of nasal congestion in children. Contains phenylpropano-lamine hydrochloride, a decongestant, and vinegar of ipecacuanha, an expectorant.

Dosage: children 6–12 years – one to two 5 ml spoonfuls; 2–6 years – one 5 ml spoonful up to four times daily. Allow four hours between doses.

CIBA

## Mycil

Double-action ointment for treating athlete's foot. Contains tolnaftate, an antifungal agent, and benzalkonium chloride, an antiseptic. Rub into infected parts morning and night. Continue treatment for at least a week after the infection has cleared. Use in conjunction with Mycil powder or spray. These contain tolnaftate and the powder contains chlorhexidine hydrochloride, an antiseptic, and can also be used to treat conditions such as prickly heat and tenderness due to excessive perspiration.

EVANS MEDICAL

## Mycota Cream and Spray

To treat athlete's foot. Cream contains the fungicides undecenoic acid and zinc undecenoate. Apply night and morning. Spray contains undecenoic acid and the fungicide dichlorophen. Also available as powder. Continue treatment for one week after all signs of infection have disappeared.     CROOKES HEALTHCARE

## Natracalm

Herbal remedy for the stress and strain of everyday life and to help disturbed nights. Tablets contain an aqueous alcoholic extract from a species of passiflora, a plant that has been used for medicinal purposes since the early nineteenth century. Take one tablet three times a day with meals. If necessary, a further tablet may be taken at bedtime.   <small>ENGLISH GRAINS HEALTHCARE</small>

## Natural Olbas Oil Inhalant Decongestant

A blend of six pure plant oils combining the essential oils of peppermint, eucalyptus, cajuput, clove, juniper berry and wintergreen with menthol. Can be used as an inhalant or to relieve muscular discomfort and rheumatic pain such as lumbago and fibrositis, sprains or pulled muscles – essential oils applied to the skin produce a feeling of warmth and a local anaesthetic action. If using as a rub, sponge painful areas with warm water if possible and dry thoroughly. Then gently and thoroughly massage Olbas Oil into the affected part. Treatment may cause perspiration.   <small>LANES</small>

## Naturest

A non-habit-forming traditional remedy for the treatment of temporary or occasional sleeplessness. Tablets contain passiflora aqu ext. – extract of passiflora, a herbal tranquilliser. Not recommended for children under 12.

Dosage: adults – two tablets three times a day after meals and up to three tablets at bedtime. If, after five days, you're still experiencing disturbed sleep, consult your medical adviser.   <small>LANES</small>

## Nelsons Arnica Cream

A topical herbal remedy traditionally used in the symptomatic treatment of bruises. Prepared from the Alpine plant *Arnica montana*. It's a healing and soothing agent when applied to bruising resulting from injuries, falls, blows and contusions. Apply gently to bruised surfaces.   <small>NELSONS</small>

## Nelsons Calendula Cream

A topical herbal remedy prepared from marigolds, traditionally used in the symptomatic treatment of sore and rough skin. Apply a little cream and rub away lightly.   <small>NELSONS</small>

## Nelsons Evening Primrose Cream

A skin cream made from the seeds of the evening primrose flower – particularly soothing when applied to dry or 'tired' skin.   <small>NELSONS</small>

## Nelsons Graphites Cream

A homoeopathic remedy for dermatitis containing sixth potency graphites – a soothing application which helps protect sensitive skin against further irritation. Apply gently to the affected area as required.                    NELSONS

## Nelsons Haemorrhoid Cream

A topical herbal remedy traditionally used in the symptomatic treatment of piles. Prepared from fresh plant tinctures including calendula and hamamelis (witch-hazel). Wash affected area with warm water and apply cream as needed.   NELSONS

## Nelsons Hay Fever Tablets

A homoeopathic remedy for the relief of hay fever with sixth homoeopathic potency of *Allium cepa, Euphrasia officinalis* and *Sabadilla officinarum*. Suck or chew two tablets at two-hourly intervals for six doses, then three times daily until symptoms subside. Children should take half the adult dose.           NELSONS

## Nelsons Rhus Tox. Cream

A topical herbal remedy traditionally used in the symptomatic treatment of rheumatic conditions. Also for strains and the effects of over-lifting. Prepared from the fresh leaves of *Rhus toxicodendron*. Massage gently into the affected area as required.                    NELSONS

## Nelsons Teething Granules

A homoeopathically prepared remedy to help bring relief from the distressing symptoms of teething. The sixth homoeopathic potency of chamomilla helps the body overcome the symptoms and may be safely taken by small infants. Tip on to a clean, dry spoon the equivalent of a pinch of granules (do not touch with the fingers). Put the granules directly into the child's mouth every two hours for up to six doses.    NELSONS

## Nelsons Travel Sickness Tablets

A homoeopathic remedy for the relief of travel sickness with sixth homoeopathic potency of Apomorph, Staphisagria, Cocculus, Theridion, Petroleum, Tabacum and Nux Vomica. Suck or chew two tablets for two hours before the journey. Take two more tablets hourly during the journey if necessary. Children should take half the adult dose.

NELSONS

## Night Cough Pastilles

Contain extract of wild cherry bark and codeine phosphate, a cough-suppressant, to relieve tickly coughs. Not suitable for children under 12. Dosage – adults may take up to four pastilles in any two-hour period, but no more than 15 in any 24-hour period.

ERNEST JACKSON

## Noctura

A homoeopathic remedy for the relief of insomnia. Contains the sixth homoeopathic potency of Kali Brom, Coffea, Passiflora, Avena Sativa, Alfalfa and Valeriana. Take two tablets four hours before retiring and two tablets at bedtime. A further two tablets may be taken during the night if required.      NELSONS

## Nupercainal

Cream containing a local anaesthetic, cinchocaine, for the relief of piles. Apply as required.      CIBA

## Nurofen

Ibuprofen tablets effective in the relief of headaches, cold and flu symptoms, rheumatic pain, muscular pain, back ache, feverishness, migraine, period pain, dental pain and neuralgia. Also available in soluble form. Not suitable for children under 12.

Dosage: initial dose two tablets with water. Then, if necessary, one or two tablets every four hours. No more than six tablets daily.

CROOKES HEALTHCARE

## Nurse Harvey's Gripe Mixture

Gripe water with dill oil, caraway oil, weak ginger tincture and the antacid sodium bicarbonate to relieve the pain of wind, tummy upsets and colic.

Dosage: children over 1 year – three to four 5 ml spoonfuls; 6–12 months – two to three 5 ml spoonfuls; 2–6 months – two 5 ml spoonfuls; 1–2 months – one 5 ml spoonful; birth to 1 month – half a 5 ml spoonful. Give one dose during or after a feed. No more than eight doses in 24 hours.      HARVEY SCRUTON

## Nylax

Laxative tablets containing phenolpthalein, powdered senna leaf and bisacodyl (a laxative). For short-term use only. Not suitable for children. One or two tablets to be taken at bedtime. A bowel movement is generally produced in 6–12 hours. Do not use during pregnancy or while breast-feeding. Do not

take if any gastro-intestinal
blockage is present.

BRITISH CHEMOTHEUTIC PRODUCTS
(EVANS MEDICAL)

## Odourless Garlic One-A-Day

Odourless garlic powder
capsules. Take one capsule
every day with water. For the
beneficial effects of garlic, see
'Herbal remedies' under COLD,
THE COMMON p.37.        EVANS

## Oil of Cloves (own brand)

An oil made from dried flower
buds which helps relieve
toothache by numbing the
sore area. To use, soak a small
piece of cotton wool and apply
to tooth. If toothache persists,
consult your dentist or doctor.

## Oilatum Emollient

A bath oil producing an
emulsion of dispersed oil in
the bath water and an even
film on the surface to aid the
treatment of dry skin
conditions. Contains liquid
paraffin, which replaces oil
and water and hydrates the
keratin – a protein in the
outer layer of the skin, and
the emulsifier wool alcohol.
Suitable for infants.

Adult's or child's bath – add
one to three capfuls to a 20-
cm deep bath of water. Soak
for 10–20 minutes. Pat dry.
Infant's bath – add half to two

capfuls to a basin of water.
Apply gently over entire body
with a sponge. Pat dry. The
oil should always be used with
water, either added to a bath
or rubbed into wet skin.   STIEFEL

## Oilatum Soap

A gentle soap with vegetable
oil to help reduce dryness. Use
as ordinary soap. Using very
little warm water, massage
rich creamy lather into the
skin with fingers or face cloth.
Rinse off, again using very
little water. Pat dry. Suitable
for infants.        STIEFEL

## Olbas Pastilles

Plant remedy for the
symptomatic relief of colds,
coughs, catarrh, sore throats,
flu, catarrhal headache and
nasal congestion. Contain
olbas oil (see NATURAL OLBAS OIL
p.184), which soothes the
throat and as pastilles dissolve
they release vapours to help
clear the head. Contain no
gelatine, so are ideal for
vegetarians and vegans.   LANES

## Opazimes

Tablets for the relief of
diarrhoea, upset stomach,
'holiday tummy' and mild
forms of gastro-enteritis.
Contain the antacid dried
aluminium hydroxide gel, as
well as light kaolin, belladonna

dry extract and morphine hydrochloride.

Dosage: adults – two tablets every four hours to a maximum of eight tablets in one 24-hour period. Children over 6 years – one tablet every four hours to a maximum of four tablets in one 24-hour period. Not to be given to infants.      RYBAR

## Optrex Clearine Eye Drops

For temporary relief of redness of the eye due to minor eye irritations such as dust, smoke and chlorine from swimming pools. Contain distilled witch-hazel to cool and naphazoline hydrochloride to relieve inflammation. For use by adults and children over 12 only. Gently squeeze one or two drops into each eye, no more than four times daily.

Not to be used by contact-lens wearers except under medical supervision. Do not use this product if you suffer from glaucoma or any serious eye disease or if you have had previous eye surgery. If you're being treated for high blood pressure, depression, heart disease, diabetes or increased thyroid activity, consult your doctor before using these drops. If you experience severe eye pain, changes of vision or discharge from the eye, or if the condition worsens or persists for more than one day, consult your doctor.      OPTREX (CROOKES HEALTHCARE)

## Optrex Eye Lotion

Gentle eye lotion with cooling witch-hazel and a small amount of the antiseptic benzalkonium chloride, to soothe tired and sore eyes. For the relief of minor eye irritations caused by dusty or smoky atmospheres, driving or close work. Also available in drop form. Not suitable for use with soft contact lenses. Always clean eye bath by boiling in water before use. Fill a third full. Do not dilute lotion. Bend head slightly forward, apply the eye bath and rock the head from side to side for at least half a minute, keeping the eyelid open so that the lotion bathes the eye's surface thoroughly. Repeat with fresh lotion to the other eye.

OPTREX (CROOKES HEALTHCARE)

## Oraldene

A solution containing hexetidine, a bactericide and fungicide, for the treatment of mouth infections such as gingivitis, chronic periodontitis, stomatitis, ulcers, bad breath and oral thrush. Also useful before and after dental surgery, in geriatric nursing and in treating tonsillitis and pharyngitis.   WARNER LAMBERT

## Otrivine
Nasal decongestant containing xylometazoline hydrochloride, available in drop or spray form for adults and children. Dosage: one application in each nostril two to three times daily. Also available as Otrivine Paediatric.   CIBA

## Ovex
Contains medendazole to treat threadworms. The tablets are orange-flavoured and may be chewed or swallowed whole. Adults and children over 2 years – take one tablet. Not suitable for children under 2.

A single tablet of Ovex will kill threadworms. However, it may not destroy the eggs, which can cause re-infection. It's therefore highly recommended that a second tablet is taken after two weeks. If you are pregnant or think you may be, do not take this product.

JANSSEN PHARMACEUTICAL

## Panadeine
Paracetamol and codeine phosphate tablets for the relief of headache, migraine, toothache, colds and flu, period pains and rheumatic pains. Not recommended for children under 7. Take with a tumblerful of water.

Dosage: adults – two tablets every four hours as needed. No more than four doses in 24 hours. Children 7–12 years – half to one tablet every four hours as needed. No more than four doses in 24 hours.

STERLING HEALTH

## Panadol and Panadol Extra
Paracetamol available in tablet, capsule or soluble form. Panadol Extra contains an additional ingredient, the stimulant caffeine. Suitable for the relief of headache, migraine, back ache, rheumatic and muscle pains, neuralgia, toothache and period pains. Also relieves discomfort in colds, flu, sore throats and helps reduce temperature. Panadol Baby and Infant Elixir and Panadol Junior (see below) can be given to children under 12. Panadol capsules and Panadol Extra should only be given to children under 12 on medical advice.

Dosage: adults – two tablets four times daily, but no more frequently than every four hours. No more than four doses in 24 hours.

STERLING HEALTH

## Panadol Junior

Paracetamol for children to relieve aches and pains such as headache, toothache, sore throat and discomfort due to colds and flu. Will also help lower raised temperature. Suitable for children aged 3–12 years. Dissolve sachet in cold water.

Dosage: children 6–12 years – one to two sachets; 3–6 years – one sachet, but for both age ranges no more than four doses in 24 hours. Do not take more frequently than at four-hourly intervals, up to the maximum daily dose.

WINPHARM (STERLING HEALTH)

## Panoxyl Aquagel 2.5, 5, 10 and Panoxyl Wash

Wash and gels for the treatment of acne. Apply once daily after washing the affected area. Contain benzoyl peroxide.                    STIEFEL

## Paracetamol (own brand)

A mild to moderate pain-reliever for the treatment of headache, migraine, neuralgia, toothache, sore throat, period pains, aches and pains, including muscle pain and backache. Also for the symptomatic relief of influenza, feverishness and feverish colds.

Dosage – generally adults and children over 12: one to two tablets every four hours. Maximum eight tablets in 24 hours. Follow instructions on label.

## Paracetamol Tablets APS

Also available in capsule form. Adults and children over 12 should take one to two tablets; children 6–12 years – half to one tablet or one capsule. Do not repeat more frequently than at four-hourly intervals and do not take more than four doses in any 24 hours.                    APS

## Paraclear and Junior Paraclear

Soluble paracetamol tablets for the relief of mild and bad headache, migraine pain, neuralgia, rheumatic and muscle pains, period pains and toothache. Also reduces temperature and relieves feverishness and the major symptoms of colds and flu. Paraclear must be taken in half a glass, or less, of water. Not suitable for children under six.

Dosage: adults – one to two tablets. No more than eight tablets in 24 hours. Children 6–12 years – half to one tablet up to four times a day. Do not repeat dose more frequently than every four hours.

Junior Paraclear – for children's painful and feverish

complaints. Soluble paracetamol tablets forming a strawberry-flavoured solution. Children 6–12 years – two to four tablets; 1-5 years – one to two tablets; 3 months to 1 year – one tablet. If necessary dose can be repeated every four hours, but do not give more than four doses in 24 hours. Do not give to children under 3 months except on a doctor's advice.  NICHOLAS

## Paracodol
Capsules and soluble tablets containing paracetamol and codeine phosphate for strong pain relief in headaches, migraine, cold and flu symptoms including raised temperature and sore throats, muscular and rheumatic pains, neuralgia, period pain and toothache. Capsules not recommended for children under 12.

Dosage: adults – one to two capsules, repeat every four to six hours if necessary, with a maximum of eight capsules in 24 hours. Soluble tablets: adults – as capsules. Children 6–12 years – half to one tablet. Repeat every six hours if necessary, with a maximum of four tablets in 24 hours.  FISONS

## Pavacol-D
Sugar-free cough mixture containing pholcodine, a cough-suppressant, for the symptomatic treatment of coughs due to upper respiratory tract infection.

Dosage: adults – one or two 5 ml spoonfuls as needed. Children 6–12 years – one 5 ml spoonful four or five times daily; 3–5 years – one 5 ml spoonful three times daily; 1–2 years – half a 5 ml spoonful three or four times daily.
BOEHRINGER INGELHEIM

## Penetrol Catarrh Lozenges
Relieve the symptoms of catarrh, hay fever and nasal congestion. Contain menthol; ammonium chloride, an expectorant; phenylephrine hydrochloride, to clear a stuffy nose; and creosote, a disinfectant. Not suitable for children under 10. Suck two, one after the other and then one every two to three hours as required.  CROOKES HEALTHCARE

## Penetrol Inhalant
Menthol and peppermint oil inhalant to relieve the symptoms of catarrh, hay fever and nasal congestion.
CROOKES HEALTHCARE

## Petrolagar
Laxative emulsion containing liquid paraffin and light liquid paraffin for the gentle relief of constipation. Adult dose – two 5 ml spoonfuls morning and night or between meals.

Reduce to an occasional dose
as required. Avoid prolonged
use.          WYETH FAMILY HEALTH

## Pholcodine Cough Pastilles
Contain pholcodine, a cough-
suppressant, to relieve a
persistent cough. Not suitable
for children under 12. Adults
should take one or two
pastilles every four hours.
          ERNEST JACKSON

## Phytocil Cream and Powder
Cream to treat athlete's foot.
Contains phenoxy-propan-2-
ol, chlorophenoxy-ethanol (an
antifungal agent), salicylic
acid, which also kills fungus,
and soothing menthol. Apply
to affected area night and
morning. Continue treatment
for at least a week after the
infection has cleared up.
Powder also contains zinc
undecenoate, an antifungal
drug, and should be used in
conjunction with the cream
for more effective relief and to
prevent re-infection.     FISONS

## Pileabs Tablets
Herbal tablets containing
powdered slippery elm bark
and cascara sagrada, a herb
with a long tradition of use in
the relief of constipation. To
help ease constipation and the
itching, irritation and
discomfort due to piles.

Gluten free. Suitable for
vegetarians.
  Directions: adults should
take two tablets with a little
water three times a day
before meals.          LANES

## Pollon-Eze
Tablets containing astemizole,
an antihistamine, sold over
the counter since 1988, for
relief from hay fever without
causing drowsiness. Adults
and children over 12 – one
tablet once a day on an empty
stomach, preferably in the
morning. If you are pregnant
or think you may be, do not
take this product. Available in
a calendar pack. Since people
vary in their response to
medications, it may take two
to three days to attain
maximum effect. For best
results, take Pollon-Eze
continuously every day for as
long as the hay-fever season
lasts.     JANSSEN PHARMACEUTICAL

## Polytar Liquid
Concentrated antiseptic tar-
medicated scalp cleanser for
the treatment of seborrhoea,
psoriasis, itching scalp and
dandruff. Contains tar, cade
oil, coal-tar solution, arachis
oil, extract of crude coal tar
and oleyl alcohol – a blend of
coal and wood tars to relieve
scaling, itching and oiliness.
It's thought that tar

compounds are able to penetrate the stratum corneum – the tough, waterproof, top layer of the skin – and slow down the division of cells.

Use as shampoo once or twice weekly, or as recommended by your doctor.

STIEFEL

## Powerin

Strong pain-relieving tablets containing aspirin, paracetamol and caffeine, for the treatment of headache, migraine, neuralgia, rheumatic, period and dental pains and the symptoms of colds and flu. Not suitable for children under 12.

Dosage – one or two tablets every four hours. No more than six in any 24 hours.

WHITEHALL

## PR Freeze Spray

Spray relief for muscular pain and stiffness, lumbago, sciatica, fibrositis, sprains and bruises. Contains trichlorofluoromethane, which has a cooling effect on the skin, and dichlorodifluoromethane, to relieve pain. Hold the can approximately 45 cm away from painful area and spray for three to five seconds. Repeat once or, if necessary, twice, at 30-second intervals.

Do not repeat this treatment more than three times a day. Do not spray on head, neck, fingers or toes. Not to be used on children under 6.

CROOKES HEALTHCARE

## PR Heat Spray

Spray relief for muscular and rheumatic pain, sprains and bruises. Works by warming the skin over the painful area. Contains the counter-irritants methyl salicylate and ethyl nicotinate, and camphor. Hold can about 15 cm away from painful area and spray two or three short bursts. Repeat up to twice daily. Spray may have a stronger effect on some people than on others, so use on a small area first. Use sparingly, as over-application can cause discomfort.

CROOKES HEALTHCARE

## Premiums

Antacid tablets containing magnesium trisilicate, dried aluminium hydroxide gel, light magnesium carbonate, creta and peppermint oil, to neutralise excess acid and give relief from heartburn, acid indigestion and sour stomach.

NEWTON CHEMICAL

## Preparation H Suppositories

Suppositories or ointment to ease the pain and irritation of piles. Use morning and night and after each bowel movement. Contains shark-liver oil and alcohol-soluble extract of live yeast cells. These work 'empirically' – that is to say, they have been found to be beneficial in some people – doctors don't really know why.                WHITEHALL

## Pripsen

Powder containing piperazine phosphate and sennosides, the main active ingredient of the laxative senna fruit, to treat threadworm and roundworm. Pripsen acts by paralysing the adult worms which are then expelled by the gentle laxative action of standardised senna.

All members of the household should be treated with Pripsen on the same day, with a follow-up dose 14 days later. This helps to ensure complete treatment of threadworm infection by eliminating those worms which were in the egg or larval stage when the first dose was given. One pack contains two sachets. The dose from one sachet should be taken at bedtime by adults and in the morning by children. Stir the contents into a small glass of milk (or water) and drink at once, any unused powder being discarded. Adults and children over 6 – one sachet. Children 1–6: two-thirds of a sachet (one level 5 ml spoonful). Infants three months to one year: consult your doctor. If you believe you may be pregnant, consult your doctor before using this product. Do not take if you have kidney disease or have ever suffered from epilepsy.

RECKITT & COLMAN

## Probase 3

Dermatological cream and lotion to moisturise dry skin conditions. Apply as often as required. Suitable for all the family.

SCHERING-PLOUGH CONSUMER HEALTH

## Proflex

Tablets containing ibuprofen for the relief of back and muscular pain. Also available in capsules designed to release slowly. Dosage, adults only: two tablets every four hours with a maximum of six in 24 hours, or one to two capsules twice a day with a maximum of four in 24 hours.        CIBA

## Propain

Analgesic tablets containing paracetamol, codeine phosphate, diphenydramine hydrochloride (an antihistamine) and caffeine. For the treatment of migraine, headache, toothache, muscular pain and period pain, and the symptomatic relief of flu, feverishness and colds. May cause drowsiness. Do not take during pregnancy or while breast-feeding.

Dosage: adults and children over 12 – one or two tablets every four hours, with not more than ten tablets in 24 hours. Avoid excessive intake of coffee or tea when taking these tablets.          PANPHARMA

## Q-Mazine Syrup

A night-time orange-flavoured syrup for the treatment of urticaria, to allow restful sleep and for prevention of travel sickness in children and babies over six months. Contains promethazine hydrochloride, an antihistamine. May cause drowsiness. Consult your pharmacist for the best use of this product.

Dosage, to be taken at bedtime: children over 5 – two to five 5 ml spoonfuls; 1–5 years – one to three 5 ml spoonfuls; 6 months to 1 year – one or two 5 ml spoonfuls. If the lower dose has been given, this may be repeated once in 24 hours but not less than six hours after the first dose.          CUPAL

## Quiet Life Tablets

Herbal remedy with no known evidence of habit-forming effects to help relieve periods of worry, irritability, stresses and strains, and to promote sleep. A blend of valerian, hops and passiflora with motherwort, wild lettuce and three B vitamins, thiamine, riboflavin and nicotinamide.          LANES

## Radian-B

A topical analgesic range containing counter-irritants to provide fast and lasting relief from muscular aches and pains. Suitable for adults and children over six. Best applied after a hot bath. The range consists of:

Radian-B Liniment containing menthol, camphor, ammonium salicylate and salicylic acid for relief over large surface areas. Massage in and repeat 10–15 minutes later. Apply up to three times a day, reducing to morning and evening when acute symptoms subside.

Radian-B Rub with menthol, camphor, methyl salicylate and capsicin (made from peppers). Massage in to ease pain.

Radian-B Spray, with the same ingredients as the liniment, but with the advantage of reaching awkward areas. Spray lightly for two to three seconds, and repeat if necessary after 10–15 minutes.

Radian-B Warm-Up
Embrocation with capsicin and methyl salicylate to warm up muscles before sport, thereby reducing the risk of injury. Massage well into the muscles.

There are also Radian-B mineral bath and mineral bath salts to soothe away aches and pains. FISONS

## Rapolyte

Oral rehydration therapy containing the essential salts and minerals sodium chloride, sodium citrate and potassium chloride. Also contains glucose. Add contents of a sachet to 200 ml fresh drinking water. For infants and if drinking water is unavailable, boil water for one minute and allow to cool. Stir well until the contents are dissolved. JANSSEN PHARMACEUTICAL

## RBC

Rybar Bite 'n' Burn soothing cream for immediate relief of insect bites, stings, nettle rash, sunburn and itching. Contains antazoline hydrochloride, an antihistamine; cetrimide, an antiseptic; and cooling calamine and camphor. Apply to affected area every three hours as necessary. If symptoms persist after two to three days, consult your doctor. RYBAR

## Regulan

Sachets containing Ispaghula husk, a miscible fibre – that means it disperses in water. Used for regulating bowel movements and softening the stools.

Dosage: adults – one or three sachets daily; children 6–12 years – half to one level 5 ml spoonful one to three times daily. PROCTER AND GAMBLE

## Reguletts

Chocolate-flavoured laxative tablets containing phenolpththalein for relieving occasional constipation. Take at bedtime for overnight action. Not suitable for children under 12. Adults and children over 12 chew one tablet carefully before swallowing. Do not take during pregnancy except on medical advice, nor while breast-feeding. CUPAL

## Rennie, Rennie Gold, Rennie Plus

Antacid tablets to relieve acid indigestion, heartburn, nervous indigestion, acidity, flatulence, upset stomach, dyspepsia or biliousness. Also available in spearmint flavour. Rennie contains calcium carbonate and light magnesium carbonate, Rennie Gold calcium carbonate. Suck or chew two tablets as needed. Repeat whenever discomfort is felt, to a maximum of 16 tablets a day for Rennie, 14 for Rennie Gold.

Rennie Plus also eases wind – it contains activated methylpolysiloxane (to break down gas), magnesium hydroxide and aluminium hydroxide/magnesium co-dried gel. Adults should suck or chew one or two tablets as needed, but not more than eight a day.                    NICHOLAS

## Resiston One

Nasal spray containing sodium cromoglycate to stop a runny nose and xylometazoline hydrochloride, a nasal decongestant, to relieve the discomfort of nasal hay-fever symptoms without causing drowsiness. Spray once into each nostril four times a day. Not suitable for children under 8. Use Resiston One continually throughout the hay-fever season for most effective defence, even when you are free of symptoms.

FISONS

## Ress Q

Pastilles containing soothing tincture of benzoin and benzalkonium chloride solution, an antiseptic, to relieve pain caused by mouth ulcers and sore gums. Adults (including the elderly) and children over 3 should dissolve one pastille in the mouth every two hours, up to a maximum of eight pastilles in any 24-hour period.

ERNEST JACKSON

## Rheumasol

A herbal medicine used for the relief of muscular pain and stiffness associated with back ache, sciatica, lumbago, fibrositis, rheumatism and painful joints. Tablets contain two plants known through the centuries for their specific action in rheumatic conditions and said to have anti-rheumatic and anti-inflammatory properties – guaiacum resin, extracted from the ornamental evergreen tree, and prickly ash bark. One tablet to be taken three times a day with meals.        ENGLISH GRAINS HEALTHCARE

## Rinstead Adult Gel

For immediate relief of mouth ulcers. Contains benzocaine, a local anaesthetic, and chloroxylenol to cover the sore area with a protective coat of soothing antiseptic. Also relieves pain from denture chafing, sore gums, cheek bites and soreness after extraction of teeth. For adults and children over 12. Apply to the sore area with a clean finger or swab up to six times a day.

SCHERING-PLOUGH CONSUMER HEALTH

## Rinstead Pastilles

Contain soothing menthol and the antiseptic chloroxylenol, to relieve pain and aid the healing of mouth ulcers. Allow one pastille to dissolve slowly in the mouth about every two hours.

SCHERING-PLOUGH CONSUMER HEALTH

## Robitussin Cough Soother

Sugar-free linctus containing dextromethorphan hydrobromide, a cough-suppressant, to relieve dry, irritating coughs without causing drowsiness.

Dosage: adults one 10 ml measure three or four times daily. Children 6–12 years, one 5 ml measure three or four times daily. Contains a sugar substitute (carbohydrate content approximately 1 gm per 5 ml) which should be safe for people with diabetes.

A.H. ROBINS

## Robitussin Cough Soother Junior

Junior version of the above, to relieve children's dry, irritating coughs without causing drowsiness. Children 6–12 years – one 10 ml measure three or four times daily; 2–6 years – one 5 ml

measure three or four times daily. Not recommended for children under 2.

A.H. ROBINS

## Robitussin Expectorant

Sugar-free expectorant containing guaiphenesin to relieve chesty coughs without causing drowsiness. Not recommended for children under 2.

Dosage to be taken four times a day. Adults – one 10 ml measure. Children 6–12 years – one 5 ml measure; 2–6 years – one 2.5 ml measure. Contains a sugar substitute (carbohydrate content approximately 1 gm per 5 ml) which should be safe for people with diabetes.

A.H. ROBINS

## Robitussin Expectorant Plus

A sugar-free expectorant linctus containing guaiphenesin and pseudoephedrine hydrochloride, a decongestant, to clear up blocked noses without causing drowsiness. Not suitable for children under 2.

Dosage, to be taken three times a day. Adults – one 10 ml measure. Children 6–12 years – one 5 ml measure; 2–6 years – one 2.5 ml measure. Contains the same sugar substitute as Robitussin Expectorant, above, so should be safe for people with diabetes.                    A.H. ROBINS

## Salatac Gel
Contains salicylic acid and lactic acid for the treatment of warts, corns and callouses. Soak the affected area in warm water for two to three minutes every night. Dry thoroughly. Apply one or two drops of gel and allow to dry. No plaster necessary. The following evening, carefully remove and discard the elastic film formed from the previous application and re-apply gel. An emery board is included in every pack to abrade stubborn warts.                    DERMAL

## Sanatogen One-A-Day Garlic Perles
Pure essential oil of garlic capsules to help support the body's natural defences. Take one capsule daily.          FISONS

## Savlon
Liquid antiseptic disinfectant and cream containing cetrimide, an antiseptic, and chlorhexidine gluconate, an antiseptic and disinfectant. Use as required.              CIBA

## Savlon Dry
Antiseptic first-aid aerosol spray for minor skin abrasions. Contains povidone iodine, an antiseptic. Use as required.              CIBA

## Savlon Nappy Rash Cream
For the treatment and prevention of nappy rash. Contains dimethicone, a water-repellant. Use as required.              CIBA

## Sea-Legs
Travel sickness tablets containing meclozine hydrochloride, an antihistamine. May cause drowsiness.

Dosage: adults and children over 12 – two tablets. Children 6–12 years – one tablet; 2–6 years – half a tablet. As Sea-Legs remain active for 24 hours, take the previous night or about one hour before the journey starts. Can also be taken for relief when you feel sickness coming on. As with all medicines, do not take during pregnancy except on medical advice.          EVANS MEDICAL

## Seldane
Tablets containing the antihistamine terfenadine to relieve symptoms of hay fever while avoiding drowsiness. One tablet lasts 24 hours. Seldane will not normally affect your ability to drive or perform tasks requiring concentration. However, as

with all drugs, care should be taken initially because there may be rare exceptions. Adults and children over 12: one tablet daily when symptoms require. Not to be used during pregnancy unless medically directed.

MERRELL DOW PHARMACEUTICALS

## Senlax

Chocolate laxative tablets with natural senna. Adults and children over 12 should take one tablet at bedtime. Children 6–12 years – half a tablet.                    INTERCARE

## Shen Garlic Tablets

Concentrated, organically grown Chinese garlic. Take one or two tablets three times a day before meals. A daily intake of six tablets provides the equivalent of an average-sized garlic clove.            LANES

## Sinex Decongestant Nasal Spray

Contains the decongestant and vasoconstrictor oxymetazoline hydrochloride and menthol, camphor and eucalyptol to clear a stuffy nose. For adults and children over 6 – at first signs of a blocked nose, spray once or twice up each nostril every six to eight hours. Do not swallow.        PROCTER AND GAMBLE

## Sinutab

Tablets containing paracetamol and phenylpropanolamine hydrochloride, a drug that constricts blood vessels to ease congestion. For the relief of sinus congestion and associated headache. Also helpful in the relief of sinus pain, fever and congestion associated with the common cold, flu and hay fever. Not suitable for children under six. Do not take during pregnancy.

Dosage: adults – two tablets three times daily. No more than six tablets in any 24-hour period. Children 6–12 years – one tablet three times daily. No more than three tablets in any 24-hour period.

WARNER LAMBERT

## Snowfire

A tablet for the treatment of chapped hands and chilblains. Contains yellow soft paraffin to moisturise and protect, and 15 natural herbal extracts including benzoin, marshmallow and thyme oil, which are all healing ingredients, and nutmeg and clove oil which bring warmth to chilblains. Wash the hands or feet in warm water, then gently rub in some of the tablet. Alternatively some of the tablet may be spread on a bandage or lint and applied to the affected area.   J. PICKLES & SONS

## Snuffle Babe

A mild vapour rub containing eucalyptus oil, menthol and thyme oil for young babies and children. The formula contains no camphor which is said to irritate the skin of young babies. Lightly rub a small amount of Snuffle Babe on to chest, throat and back. Leave bed coverings loose so that beneficial vapours emitted may be inhaled during the night. Keep away from eyes. Do not use on infants' nostrils. For external use only.

J. PICKLES & SONS

## Solarcaine

Lotion containing the local anaesthetic benzocaine and antiseptic triclosan for relief from the pain of sunburn and for general first aid – cuts, bites, scratches and minor burns. Apply freely to the skin. Limit use to three to four times daily. Not suitable for children under 3. Not for deep or puncture wounds or serious burns nor for prolonged or extensive use.

SCHERING-PLOUGH CONSUMER HEALTH

## Solmin

Tablets containing aspirin which disperse on the tongue without water for the relief of mild to moderate pain in headaches, including tension and migraine headaches, toothache, neuralgia, period pains, rheumatic pain, lumbago and sciatica. Also relieves the symptoms of influenza, feverishness and feverish colds, and eases sore throats. Adults and children over 12: one to three tablets every four hours. No more than 13 tablets to be taken in any 24-hour period. Not to be given to children under 12 except on a doctor's advice.

RECKITT & COLMAN

## Solpadeine

Strong pain relief in soluble tablets or capsules containing paracetamol, codeine phosphate and caffeine. For treatment of migraine, headache, rheumatic pain, period pains, toothache, neuralgia, colds, flu, sore throat and feverishness. Capsules not suitable for children under 12. Tablets not for children under 7. Tablets should be dissolved in a tumblerful of water.

Dosage: adults – two tablets or capsules up to four times daily. No more than eight in 24 hours. Children 7–12 years – half to one tablet up to four times daily, not more often than every four hours. No more than four tablets in 24 hours.

Do not give Solpadeine to children for more than three days without consulting a doctor.          STERLING HEALTH

## Soothene Ointment

An antiseptic ointment containing methyl salicylate, camphor and zinc oxide, with a blend of witch-hazel, eucalyptus oil and ti-tree oil. For the treatment of scratches, stings, chilblains, spots, pimples and other common skin problems.     LANES

## Strepsils

Throat lozenges for adults and children, available in original flavour, honey and lemon, Vitamin C and menthol and eucalyptus. Contain two antiseptics, dichlorobenzyl alcohol and amylmetacresol. Dissolve one lozenge slowly in the mouth every two to three hours.

CROOKES HEALTHCARE

## Stugeron

Travel-sickness tablets containing cinnarizine, an antihistamine. May cause drowsiness. Tablets may be sucked, chewed or swallowed.

Dosage: adults and children over 12 – two tablets two hours before travelling. One further tablet every eight hours as needed. Children 5–12 years – one tablet two hours before travelling. A further half-tablet every eight hours as needed.

JANSSEN PHARMACEUTICAL

## Sudafed.Co

Tablets containing paracetamol and the decongestant pseudoephedrine hydrochloride to relieve cold and flu symptoms such as aches and pains, feverishness, blocked-up nose and sinuses, without causing drowsiness.

Dosage: adults and children over 12 – one tablet three times a day. Children 6–12 years – half a tablet three times a day. Safety advice as for Sudafed Expectorant, below.          WELLCOME

## Sudafed Expectorant

Contains guaiphenesin and pseudoephedrine hydrochloride to fight congestion. To loosen stubborn mucus, clear chesty coughs and help relieve the symptoms of nasal congestion such as blocked sinuses, stuffed-up nose or catarrh. Does not cause drowsiness.

Dosage, to be taken three times a day. Adults and children over 12 – two 5 ml spoonfuls. Children 6–12 years – one 5 ml spoonful; 2–5 years – half a 5 ml spoonful.

As with all medicines, if you're pregnant or currently taking any other medicine, consult your doctor or pharmacist before taking this product.

WELLCOME

## Sudafed Elixir
A mixture containing the decongestant pseudoephedrine hydrochloride to relieve colds and flu symptoms such as blocked sinuses, stuffed-up nose and catarrh without causing drowsiness. Dosage and safety advice as for Sudafed Expectorant, above.

WELLCOME

## Sudafed Linctus
Contains dextromethorphan hydrobromide, a cough-suppressant, and the decongestant pseudoephedrine hydrochloride, to soothe and control dry coughs and help relieve the symptoms of nasal congestion such as blocked sinuses, stuffed-up nose and catarrh. Dosage and safety advice as for Sudafed Expectorant, above, but also avoid alcoholic drink.　WELLCOME

## Sudafed Tablets
Contain the decongestant pseudoephedrine hydrochloride to relieve cold and flu symptoms such as blocked sinuses, stuffed-up nose and catarrh without

causing drowsiness. Adults and children over 12 only – one tablet three times a day.

WELLCOME

## Sudocrem
An antiseptic healing cream for the treatment of cuts and grazes, nappy rash, sunburn, acne, eczema, bed sores, chilblains and minor burns. Contains the antiseptics benzyl alcohol and benzyl benzoate, skin protectors zinc oxide and lanolin, and preservative benzyl cinnamate.　TOSARA

## Suleo-C Carbaryl Lotion
A two-hour treatment lotion containing carbaryl to kill head lice. Keeping head upright, rub the lotion well in until scalp and all hair is thoroughly moistened. This could take up to one bottle per head. If applying to a child, hold a towel to the forehead to protect the eyes. Allow hair to dry naturally in a well-ventilated room. Don't use a hairdryer. After two hours, shampoo in normal manner with an ordinary shampoo. A hairdryer may now be used.

Used as directed, a single application of this lotion will kill both head lice and their eggs within two hours. Not to be used on infants less than six months old except under medical supervision.

INTERNATIONAL LABORATORIES

## Suleo-C Carbaryl Shampoo

Contains carbaryl to eradicate head lice infection. Treatment should consist of three shampoo applications at intervals of three days. Use as normal shampoo, but leave second lather on head for five minutes. Rinse off with clean water. Comb out hair with a fine-toothed comb and then dry.

INTERNATIONAL LABORATORIES

## Suleo-M Malathion Lotion

A two-hour treatment lotion to kill head lice. Use as directed for Suleo-C Carbaryl Lotion, above.

INTERNATIONAL LABORATORIES

## Sun E45

From the makers of Cream E45 (see p.150), a perfume-free range containing titanium dioxide, a non-irritant sunscreen, that gives protection against UVA and UVB rays, while allowing a gradual tan. For children and adults with sun-sensitive skin.

The range includes UVA/UVB sun block cream SPF25 – for fair skin types, children and adults who always burn and never tan. Ultra UVA/UVB Protection Lotion for children and adults who always burn and sometimes tan. High UVA/UVB Protection Lotion for people who sometimes burn, but will tan and want to take care of their skin.

Sun E45 is long-lasting and water-resistant, so it doesn't require frequent re-application – every three hours is usually enough, unless you rub it off while towelling yourself dry.

CROOKES HEALTHCARE

## Sure-Lax

Raspberry-flavoured laxatives containing yellow phenolphthalein. Dosage: adults – one tablet to be chewed at bedtime. Children over 8 – half a tablet at bedtime.

THOMAS GUEST

## Syndol

Tablets specially formulated to relieve tension headache. Syndol contains paracetamol, codeine phosphate and doxylamine succinate (an antihistamine) and the stimulant caffeine. Adults and children 12 years and older: take one or two tablets every four or six hours as needed for relief. Do not exceed eight tablets per day. Syndol tablets should not be taken continuously over prolonged periods in the maximum dose.

Do not exceed the stated dose.
May cause drowsiness.

## Teejel Gel

A sugar-free gel for the relief
of pain in teething. Can also
be used to treat mouth ulcers,
denture irritation and cold
sores. Contains an antiseptic,
cetalkonium chloride, and an
analgesic, choline salicylate,
which is closely related to
aspirin but is more soluble,
enabling it to be absorbed
through the mucosa of the
mouth and other parts of the
body. The gel shouldn't be
used if a baby is being
prescribed, or is allergic to,
aspirin.                          NAPP

## Throaties

Range of pastilles. Throaties
Originals contain soothing
benzoin tincture and menthol
for chest and throat relief for
the symptoms of coughs and
colds. Throaties Blackcurrant
Flavour Pastilles and
Throaties Lemon, Honey and
Menthol Flavour soothe
minor throat irritations and
ease dry tickling coughs.
Blackcurrant Flavour contains
honey, ascorbic acid and
menthol. Lemon contains
honey, lemon oil and menthol.
May be taken with reasonable
freedom.

Throaties Catarrh Pastilles,
for the relief of catarrh
symptoms with congestion,
contain easing menthol,
abietis pine oil, sylvestris pine
oil and creosote, a disinfectant.
Dosage for adults and children
over 12 – no more than 20
pastilles in 24 hours. Children
6–12 years – no more than 12
pastilles in 24 hours.

Throaties Extra are pastilles
for the relief of sore throats
and the symptoms of
bronchial catarrh, coughs and
colds. Contain soothing
benzoin tincture, menthol and
aniseed oil. Dissolve one
pastille slowly in the mouth
when required.

Other soothing pastilles
from the same manufacturer
include Liquorice and Aniseed
Lozenges, Honey and Rosehip
Lozenges, Menthol and
Eucalyptus Lozenges,
Proctor's Pinelyptus Pastilles
(for loss of voice, relief of
husky voice, minor throat
irritations and coughs),
Glycerine Thymol Pastilles
(for sore throats), Lemon,
Glycerine and Honey Pastilles,
Blackcurrant and Glycerine
Pastilles, Glycerine and
Natural Oil of Lemon
Pastilles, Lemon and Lime
Pastilles, Pine and Eucalyptus
Pastilles (to relieve a husky
voice) and Cough Pastilles
with Eucalyptus and Menthol.

There is also a range of sugar-free fruit pastilles.   ERNEST JACKSON

## Tinaderm Powder
Contains tolnaftate to treat athlete's foot and other fungal infections of the skin, particularly in moist areas. Especially recommended for use on areas where perspiration is a problem. Dust affected area night and morning. A sprinkling of powder daily inside socks or stockings will help prevent athlete's foot. Tinaderm Solution is also available and the two products may be used together.

SCHERING-PLOUGH CONSUMER HEALTH

## Tineafax Cream and Powder
Soothing treatment containing tolnaftate, providing relief from athlete's foot and other minor fungal infections of the skin. Use cream night and morning. Reduce to one treatment daily as healing progresses. Use powder frequently in conjunction with cream, at least twice daily.   WELLCOME

## Tixylix
Blackcurrant-flavoured children's cough linctus to relieve troublesome, tickly coughs. Contains promethazine hydrochloride, an antihistamine, and pholcodine, a cough-suppressant. Also eases sore throats, runny and blocked-up noses. May cause drowsiness. Aids restful sleep. Use the measuring cup provided to give doses two to three times a day. Children 6–10 years – 5–10 ml; 3–5 years – 5 ml; 1–2 years – 2.5ml.   INTERCARE

## Tramil 500
Paracetamol capsules for the treatment of headache, migraine, neuralgia, rheumatic, period and dental pains and the symptoms of colds and flu. Not suitable for children under six.

Dosage: adults – two capsules every four hours. Children 6–12 years – half the adult dose. Maximum eight capsules (children four capsules) in any 24-hour period.   WHITEHALL

## Tri-Ac
Face-wash lotion and gel treatments and preventatives for acne. Lotion and gel contain ethyl lactate, a mild antiseptic, and zinc sulphate, an astringent. Use as required.

CIBA

## Triludan and Triludan Forte
Tablets containing the antihistamine terfenadine for the effective treatment of hay

fever, rhinitis, insect bites and nettle rashes while avoiding drowsiness. Triludan will not normally affect your ability to drive or perform tasks requiring concentration. However, as with all drugs, care should be taken initially because there may be rare exceptions.

Dosage – adults and children over 12: one tablet twice daily (or two tablets together in the morning if preferred). Children 6–12: half a tablet twice daily.

Triludan Forte contains a higher dose of terfenadine. Adults and children over 12 should take one tablet in the morning. Neither form of Triludan should be taken during pregnancy unless medically directed.    MERRELL DOW

## Triogesic
Decongestant (phenylpropanolamine hydrochloride) and analgesic (paracetamol) tablets to clear nasal and sinus congestion and the headache and pain that accompany colds and sinusitis. Not recommended for children under 6. Not to be taken during pregnancy or while breast-feeding.

Dosage, to be taken up to four times daily, leaving at least four hours between doses: adults and children over

12 – one to two tablets. Children 6-12 – one tablet.
INTERCARE

## Triominic
Decongestant cold and allergy relief tablets containing pheniramine maleate, an antihistamine, and phenylpropanolamine hydrochloride, a decongestant. Not recommended for children under 6. Not to be taken during pregnancy or while breast-feeding.

Dosage, to be taken up to four times a day, leaving at least four hours between doses: adults and children over 12 – one tablet. Children 6–12 years – half a tablet.    INTERCARE

## Tyrocane
Colour-free, sugar-free throat lozenges containing the antiseptic cetylpyridinium and the antibiotic tyrothricin with the local anaesthetic benzocaine, for the relief of pain and minor infections in the mouth and throat. Not suitable for children under 12. Adults (including the elderly) and children over 12 may suck one lozenge every three or four hours as needed. Do not take more than seven lozenges a day or 15 lozenges in three days.    CUPAL

### Tyrocane Junior Antiseptic Lozenges
Sugar-free, orange-flavoured lozenges containing the antiseptic cetylpyridinium chloride to help fight against infections in the throat and nose. Not suitable for children under 6. One lozenge to be sucked slowly as needed. Do not take more than eight lozenges in one day.                   CUPAL

### Tyrozets
Aniseed-flavoured lozenges for minor mouth and throat irritations, secondary irritation following a tonsillectomy and other mouth and throat surgery. Contains an antibiotic, tyrothricin, and a local anaesthetic, benzocaine. Not recommended for children under 3. Adults should dissolve one lozenge slowly in the mouth every three hours, with a maximum of eight lozenges in 24 hours. Reduce dosage for children. Do not use for longer than five consecutive days.
                   MERCK, SHARP AND DOHME

### Ulc-Aid
Sugar-free soothing throat lozenges for mouth ulcers and sore throat. Contain tyrothricin, an antibacterial agent; benzocaine, a local anaesthetic; and cetylpyridinium chloride, an antiseptic. Not suitable for children under 12. Adults (including the elderly) and children over 12 – suck one lozenge slowly every three or four hours as required. Do not take more than seven lozenges a day or 15 lozenges in three days.                   CUPAL

### Ulc-Aid Gel
Contains an antiseptic, cetylpyridinium chloride, and a local anaesthetic, lignocaine hydrochloride, for the treatment of mouth ulcers. Suitable for adults and children. Apply a little gel to the ulcer with a clean fingertip or swab. May be repeated after 20 minutes and then every three hours if necessary. Not suitable for treating teething problems in babies.                   CUPAL

### Uvistat
Sun-protection range that protects against both UVA and UVB rays. Products contain the sunscreens mexenone, ethyl hexyl p-methoxycinnamate and butyl methoxydibenzoylmethane. Some also contain micronised titanium dioxide, a reflectant sunscreen.

Uvistat Babysun Factor 12 and 22 protect young skin. Both are water-resistant. Factor 22 should be used on fair-skinned and very young children, while Factor 12 is ideal for older children to build a tan gradually while helping to protect the skin from sun damage.

The adult Uvistat range provides protection from Factor 20 (high-protection sunblock) to Factor 4 (low-protection sun cream). Uvistat Lipscreen Factor 15 is also available.   WINDSOR PHARMACEUTICALS

## Valderma range

Valderma Active Gel contains benzoyl peroxide to treat more stubborn spots and acne. Apply once or twice daily to the whole of the affected areas. Very fair-skinned people should apply gel cautiously for the first few days. Continue daily treatment while spots persist, then apply two or three times a week to help keep skin clear.

Valderma Antibacterial Cream contains potassium hydroxyquinoline sulphate, an antibacterial agent, and chlorocresol, an antiseptic, for the treatment of everyday spots. Use two or three times a day, especially at night and in the morning.

Valderma Antibacterial Soap contains trichlorocarbanilide, an antibacterial agent, to help keep skin clear, clean and free

from spots. Also contains lanolin to soften and smooth the surface of the skin. Use at least twice daily, as oil and dirt soon build up again, even while you are asleep.   ROCHE

## Vapex

Inhalant containing menthol for relief from colds and nasal catarrh. Sprinkle a few drops on your handkerchief, then inhale vapour deeply and often during the day. At night a drop on your pillow acts while you sleep.   FISONS

## Veganin

Tablets containing paracetamol, aspirin and codeine phosphate for the relief of the symptoms of flu and all kinds of mild to moderate pain especially headache, period pain, rheumatism and toothache. Not suitable for children under 12.

Dosage: adults – one or two tablets to be swallowed every three or four hours up to a maximum of eight tablets in 24 hours.   WARNER LAMBERT

## Vicks Chloraseptic Sore Throat Lozenges

Lozenges with same anaesthetic action as Vicks Sore Throat Spray (see below). Contain phenol, a disinfectant, and sodium phenolate. Not suitable for children under 6 unless directed by a doctor.

Dosage: adults – dissolve one lozenge in the mouth every two hours. No more than eight in any 24-hour period. Children 6–12 years – one lozenge every three hours. No more than four in any 24-hour period.

PROCTER AND GAMBLE

## Vicks Chloraseptic Sore Throat Spray
Contains phenol and sodium phenolate to relieve sore throat pain. Adults – spray back of throat five times. Repeat every two hours as needed. Children under 12 – use only when recommended by a doctor. Can also be used as a gargle and mouthwash. If you have difficulty in breathing, noisy breathing or severe difficulty in swallowing, stop using this product and consult your doctor.     PROCTER AND GAMBLE

## Vicks ColdCare
Cold-treatment capsules containing paracetamol to relieve aches and pains and bring down temperature; dextromethorphan hydrobromide, a cough-suppressant; and phenylpropanolamine hydrochloride, to ease

congestion without causing drowsiness.

Dosage: adults and children over 12 – two capsules every four hours, maximum of eight in 24 hours. Children 6–12 years – one capsule every four hours, maximum of four in 24 hours. If you're under the care of your doctor or receiving continual prescribed medication or if you are pregnant, consult your doctor before using this product.

PROCTER AND GAMBLE

## Vicks Cough Syrup Expectorant
Syrup to help loosen and ease chesty coughs. Contains guaiphenesin, an expectorant; cetylpyridinium chloride, an antiseptic; and sodium citrate.

Dosage: adults over 12 – two 5 ml spoonfuls. Children 6–12 years – one 5ml spoonful. To be repeated every three hours as needed.

PROCTER AND GAMBLE

## Vicks Vapo-Lem
Hot natural lemon cold and flu remedy with Vicks vapours. Contains paracetamol to ease headache and other aches and pains, and lower temperature; phenylephrine hydrochloride to clear a stuffy nose; and ascorbic acid (Vitamin C). Not to be taken by children under

6 except on medical advice.

Dosage: adults and children over 12 – pour contents of one sachet into a tumbler and fill with hot water. Sweeten to taste. Repeat every four hours if necessary, no more than six doses in 24 hours. Children 6–12 years – half adult dose.        PROCTER AND GAMBLE

## Vicks Vapo Rub

Vapour rub decongestant for colds. Contains menthol, camphor, turpentine oil, eucalyptus, nutmeg, cedar wood oils and thymol. Use at first sign of a cold to get maximum benefit.

Children and adults – rub liberally on to chest, throat and back – cover whole area for maximum effect. Apply especially at bedtime. Leave nightclothes loose to allow vapours to be inhaled easily. For babies (over six months) apply lightly to chest and back. Rub in gently.

Can also be used as an inhalant.        PROCTER AND GAMBLE

## Vicks Vaposyrup for Dry Coughs

Contains dextromethorphan hydrobromide, a cough-suppressant, for dry coughs and a cough-irritated throat. Not suitable for children under six.

Dosage: adults and children over 12 – three 5 ml spoonfuls. Children 6–12 years – one 5 ml spoonful. Repeat every six hours as needed. No more than four doses a day.        PROCTER AND GAMBLE

## Wash E45

A washing cream for cleansing dry, sensitive and irritated skin. Free from perfume, soap and detergents. Contains a blend of mineral oils and zinc oxide to help the skin retain natural moisture. Use on face or body, wherever skin feels dry. Apply direct on to dry skin, even before a bath or shower. Massage lightly and rinse off. Take care not to slip. And, as with soap, avoid contact with the eyes.

CROOKES HEALTHCARE

## Wasp-Eze

Spray relief from stings – wasp stings, mosquito bites, nettle stings, bee stings, jellyfish stings, ant bites. Contains the antihistamine mepyramine maleat and the local anaesthetic benzocaine. Stings should be removed if possible.

Hold spray very close to skin (about 5 mm away). Spray affected area until all pain has gone – this may take up to five seconds. Repeat once after 15 minutes if necessary. Do not apply to broken skin or use near eyes.

Mosquito bites sometimes produce reactions several hours later. If symptoms persist or worsen, consult your doctor.

INTERNATIONAL LABORATORIES

## Witch Doctor

Antiseptic and astringent natural witch-hazel gel formulation to soothe skin irritation, bruises, itching, insect bites, stings, sunburn and minor burns. Squeeze gel directly on to affected area. Leave to dry. Do not use in eyes. Also available in solid form – Witch Stik.          ETHICHEM

## Zam-Buk Medicated Ointment

Contains eucalyptus oil, camphor, thyme oil and colophony (made from pine oils) to aid gentle healing of minor cuts and grazes, chapped hands, chilblains, sore aching feet. To treat minor cuts and grazes – bathe gently, apply ointment lightly, use a dressing. For chapped hands and chilblains – rub gently into the affected area. For aching feet – bathe feet in warm water, then rub in ointment. Discontinue use and consult your doctor if excessive irritation or inflammation develops. People with delicate skin may react to the ingredients in this product.          FISONS

## Zensyls

Lime-flavoured antiseptic throat therapy in a lozenge. Contains benzalkonium chloride solution. Suitable for adults and children over 5. Dissolve one lozenge slowly in the mouth as required.

ERNEST JACKSON

# Vitamins, Minerals and Supplements

## VITAMINS

Vitamins are an essential part of your diet – and as long as you eat a well-balanced diet, remembering that the fresher the food, the higher the vitamin content, you should get all the vitamins you need. The exception to this rule is Vitamin D, which is created in our skin when we are exposed to sunshine. But the simple fact that vitamins are readily available in fresh food doesn't seem to prevent us spending more and more money each year on vitamins – the figure reached £81 million in 1990!

One of the reasons for this could be that today's busy lifestyles mean we don't always eat the sort of food we ought to, and bad habits can make things worse – smoking, for instance, depletes the body of Vitamins B6, B12, C and E. On the other hand, with our generally raised consciousness about healthy eating, we know that we need vitamins and, to make sure we get them, many of us like to take supplements. Children, growing rapidly, have a greater demand for some vitamins than adults and many parents choose to give supplements in order to guarantee that their children have enough, especially if they are fussy eaters.

### Vitamin A

Essential for growth, strong bones and teeth in children, Vitamin A raises resistance to infections, aids healing, promotes tooth and skin health and is needed for night vision. It's now thought that an excessive intake of Vitamin A in pregnancy may lead to birth defects.

Vitamin A comes in two forms – retinol and carotene. Carotene is found in green vegetables and in red/orange-coloured foods like peaches,

apricots and carrots, but has
to be converted into retinol in
the body. Other good sources
of Vitamin A include liver,
kidney, milk (although semi-
skimmed and skimmed
contain much less), egg yolk,
butter and margarine.

Supplements available:
Totavit Halibut Liver Oil
Capsules (Cupal)

## The B Vitamins
The three main B vitamins –
thiamin (B1), niacin, and
riboflavin (B2) – work
together to release energy
from food. They also help
maintain the health of our
digestion, skin and nervous
system.

Good sources of thiamin
include cereals, egg yolk, fresh
pineapple, peanuts,
wheatgerm, kidney and liver;
sources of riboflavin are liver,
milk, brewers' yeast powder,
cottage cheese, poultry and
mushrooms; and of niacin,
meat and green leafy
vegetables.

Vitamin B5, pantothenic
acid, helps cortisone release
and increases energy. Good
sources include beans, chick
peas, nuts, egg yolks, avocado
pears, royal jelly.

Vitamin B6 – pyridoxine – is
essential to help the body
convert protein so that it can
use it; it also promotes health
of skin, nerves and muscle.
Good sources are meat, fish,
wholemeal foods, milk,
cabbage, yeast and
wheatgerm. Some women
find B6 helpful in overcoming
pre-menstrual syndrome, of
which common physical
symptoms are headaches, a
general feeling of bloatedness
and tenderness in the breasts.
Emotional symptoms include
weepiness, forgetfulness,
anxiety or depression and bad
temper. It's suggested that
you take Vitamin B6 three
days before problems are
expected and continue
throughout your period.
Some women also claim that
B6 supplements have helped
reduce nausea in pregnancy.

Vitamin B12 is vital for cell
formation and is important in
the production of red blood
cells. Good sources include
dairy produce, fish,
wheatgerm, beef and pork.

Folic acid, another of the
Vitamin B complex, is
essential for growth and blood
formation. There's evidence to
suggest that it might help
prevent spina bifida if taken
by women before conception,
although there's some
disagreement over this. Good
sources are offal, green
vegetables, oranges, eggs,
yeast and cereals.

Supplements available:

Benerva Compound Vitamin B, Becosyn Forte Vitamin B Complex and Berocca Effervescent Vitamin B Group (Roche); Golden Health Vitamin B Complex (English Grains); Sanatogen Vitamin B Complex; Vitamin B Complex (Evans); Benadon Vitamin B6 50 mg (Roche); Golden Health Vitamin B6 (English Grains); Sanatogen Vitamin B6 50 mg; Vitamin B6 50 mg capsules (Evans)

## Vitamin C

Essential for the health of cells, blood vessels, gums and teeth, for the healing of wounds and to help absorb iron from food. Also needed for connective tissue in skin, ligaments and bone.

It's argued that Vitamin C supplements can help replace the Vitamin C used up rapidly as the body fights colds and flu, and therefore help maintain good health. There is no convincing evidence that large doses of Vitamin C will prevent colds, but many people take it in the belief that it will. Fortunately, Vitamin C is one of the vitamins that can safely be taken in larger doses than are required for the body's everyday needs.

It is water-soluble and can be lost during cooking. Oxidation also causes loss of Vitamin C in food that is kept hot – in canteens, for instance.

Good sources include blackcurrants, oranges, new potatoes, strawberries and green leafy vegetables.

Supplements available: Centurion Vitamin C Pastilles (Ernest Jackson); Golden Health Vitamin C (English Grains); Redoxon Vitamin C 50 mg tablets (Roche); Redoxon Chewable Vitamin C 500 mg (orange- or blackcurrant-flavoured tablets from Roche); Redoxon Effervescent Vitamin C 1000 mg (lemon- or lime-flavoured tablets from Roche); Sanatogen Chewable Vitamin C 30 mg, and Vitamin High C 500 mg.

## Vitamin D

Needed to absorb the calcium from food necessary for healthy teeth and bones. Lack of Vitamin D causes rickets – poor bone formation – in children, and adults may suffer from loss of calcium in the bones – osteomalacia.

Good sources include cod-liver oil, oily fish, butter, milk, egg yolk, chicken and beef liver.

Supplements available: Cod-Liver Oil Capsules (for Vitamins A and D – Evans); Crookes Halibut-Liver Oil Capsules (Vitamins A and D);

Golden Health Cod-Liver Oil (English Grains); Sanatogen Natural Cod-Liver Oil Liquid or Capsules; Totavit Cod-Liver Oil Capsules (for Vitamins A and D – Cupal)

## Vitamin E

Also known as tocopherol and 'the vitality vitamin', Vitamin E protects the fats that are part of the structure of all cells and is vital for healthy cell structure. It protects the lungs and other tissues from damage by pollutants. It's been suggested that it may be necessary for development and maintenance of healthy red blood cells, smooth muscle, skin and other tissues. Good sources include vegetable oils, wholemeal bread, wholegrain cereals, egg yolks, nuts and green vegetables.

Supplements available: Crookes Wheatgerm Oil Capsules; Ephynal Vitamin E 50 mg (Roche); Golden Health Vitamin E (English Grains); Sanatogen Vitamin E 400 iu; Vitamin E 200 iu (Evans)

Multivitamin supplements available: Crookes Multivitamins without Iron and Multivitamins with Iron; Golden Health Children's Multivitamins A, C and D and Multivitamins and Iron (English Grains); Haliborange Orange, Blackcurrant and Multivitamin; Haliborange Multivitamin Orange Flavour Liquid; Multivitamins and Multivitamins Plus Iron (Evans); Sanatogen Multivitamins, Multivitamins and Iron, Childplan 3–5 years and 6–12 years and Children's Vitamins (A, C and D); Supradyn Ten Multivitamins for Children (Roche); Vitabites Children's Chewable Vitamins A, C and D (English Grains)

## MINERALS

As with vitamins, whether or not mineral supplements are required to maintain the health of an adult eating a regular, average diet is still open to doubt. However, doctors will prescribe supplements of iron, for example, to those groups at special risk of developing a deficiency at certain times in their lives – pregnant women and the elderly, for instance. Vitamins and minerals are also recommended medically for some children and nursing mothers. For an iron deficiency anaemia, the prescription of iron will usually be essential, as will Vitamin B12 for macrocytic anaemia.

Vitamins receive a lot of publicity and most people now know something about their benefits. However, comparatively few people know much about minerals. Some of their names will be familiar, though. Calcium, sodium (salt), iron and iodine, for instance, are commonly known to be a necessary part of a healthy diet.

The idea of eating minerals may not sound very appetising, but of course we actually absorb them without realising it from a wide range of everyday foods. Some foods are richer in minerals than others, but much depends on the mineral content of the soil in which grains, fruit, nuts and vegetables are grown and, in the case of meat and fish, the mineral content of the foods which the animals themselves have eaten.

Modern farming methods, the widespread use of fertilisers and pollution of the environment have depleted the mineral content of the soil. Food-processing and refining also remove valuable minerals and we may only absorb a small proportion of the minerals we do eat. Add the fact that many people are eating less in order to control their weight and it is easy to

see why lack of minerals may be fairly common.

## Calcium

Helps build and maintain healthy bones and teeth. Because our bones are continually building and remodelling themselves, we all need calcium throughout our lives, even when our bodies stop growing. Up until our mid twenties we can increase the amount of calcium in our bones, but after this age women especially start to lose more than can be replaced. Recent medical evidence suggests that an adequate intake of calcium early in life can help to limit this loss.

Often in our attempts to eat less fat these days we may also be cutting down on calcium, which is found in certain foods with a higher fat content. Calcium is absorbed more effectively in the presence of Vitamin D.

## Iron

Important for physical strength, stamina and mental alertness.

## Trace Elements

Other less well known but equally essential minerals include phosphorus, magnesium, manganese, zinc, chromium, copper and selenium.

The good news is that only a tiny regular amount of each of the minerals is needed to keep us healthy; in fact some (iodine, iron, zinc and selenium, for example) are known as trace elements because the amount required is so minute – though nonetheless essential.

Not all deficiency symptoms are as dramatic as those of lack of iodine – the development of a goitre and underfunctioning of the thyroid gland – but more and more evidence is emerging that many common ailments may be caused or aggravated by prolonged deficiency of one or more of the essential minerals and that correct daily intake can have a protective and preventive effect upon our health.

Some research has shown that two minerals in particular – zinc and selenium – have a beneficial effect upon our immune (disease-fighting) system. Zinc-containing lozenges, sucked every two hours during the day while symptoms last, are suggested to shorten the usual duration of a cold. Studies indicate that adequate daily amounts of selenium can protect against heart disease, relieve arthritis

and possibly slow down the ageing process.

Another study shows that a deficiency of selenium in the diet increases the risk of developing cancer. So how much do we need? The British soil (except in parts of Norfolk) is particularly lacking in selenium. It is estimated that the average diet in this country provides about 60 micrograms a day and that our daily requirement is around 200 micrograms. So it would seem a wise precaution to take a daily supplement. Selenium, to be effective, must be taken with Vitamin E. Vitamins A and C are also thought to increase its benefits.

Minerals interact with each other in our body and too much of one can inhibit the action of another. Taking supplements should therefore be approached cautiously so that the right balance is achieved – seek your pharmacist's advice if in doubt.

Multivitamin and Mineral Supplements available: Larkhall Natural Health produce a vast range of vitamins, minerals and food supplements under the brand names Cantassium, Trufree and Aquamaid.

Wassen International

produce Selenium ACE – formulated for the middle-aged and elderly; Magnesium OK – for women from 16 upwards; Confiance – for women at the menopause and onwards; Genesis for men and women from 16 upwards; Pollen B; Sitosterol-B for all ages.

Other supplements available include: Calcia, a calcium, iron and vitamin supplement especially formulated for women (English Grains); Golden Health Calcium with Vitamins A and D (English Grains); Sanatogen Multivitamins and Calcium; Supradyn Multivitamins with Minerals (capsules or effervescent tablets containing 12 vitamins and eight minerals, from Roche); Totavit Multivitamins and Minerals Capsules (eight vitamins and three minerals from Cupal). Seven Seas also produce a wide range of vitamins and minerals.

# OTHER SUPPLEMENTS

There is now a whole range of other supplements appearing more frequently on the pharmacy and health-shop shelves. These include oil of evening primrose, fish oils, ginseng and royal jelly supplements.

## Oil of Evening Primrose

The very words have a soothing ring to them and indeed the old herbal name for the evening primrose was 'king's cure all'. Although we should not take this too literally, scientific studies are beginning to show that the oil does have healing and protective properties and may relieve conditions as diverse as arthritis, eczema, premenstrual syndrome, circulatory disorders and even multiple sclerosis.

It seems that the magic ingredient of the oil is an essential fatty acid, gamma linolenic acid – GLA for short. This is not normally available in our diet (except in human breast milk), but is produced in the body and in turn is needed for the body to form prostaglandins, substances which have a wide range of beneficial effects – they can reduce inflammation, lower blood pressure, help prevent thrombosis (blood-clotting) and aid the immune (disease-fighting) system. As we age, our body's natural production of GLA may diminish because of illness, stress and other factors. To guard against a deficiency, a supplement of evening primrose oil will provide a direct supply of GLA.

Supplements available: Evening Primrose Oil 500 mg (Evans); Golden Health Evening Primrose Oil (English Grains); Sanatogen Evening Primrose Oil enriched with Oil of Borage 250 mg

## Fish Oils

Every three minutes someone dies of heart disease in the UK – that amounts to 200,000 people every year. We would all like to avoid a heart attack, if possible, and it seems that the Japanese and the Eskimos – who eat a lot of fish and rarely suffer from heart attacks – may have the answer.

This unique protection from fish oils comes from essential fatty acids called EPA (eicosapentaenoic acid) and DHA (docosahexaenoic acid), part of a group called Omega-3. Studies of EPA and DHA have shown that they decrease production of substances involved in causing inflammation and thrombosis as well as lowering the level of blood fats. The reduction of blood fat levels also reduces the risk of arteriosclerosis (the narrowing and hardening of the arteries that supply the heart muscle with blood).

Supplements available: Haliborange Fish Oil Tablets; Sanatogen Omega-3 Capsules; Pulse Pure Fish Oils

## Ginseng

Otherwise known as the 'Root of Life', this is the root of a plant which has been used in the Far East for more than 5,000 years. It is said to contain beneficial organic acids, vitamins, minerals, enzymes and amino acids which are thought to build up general vitality and increase energy. It is also thought to increase blood pressure – so caution is necessary in those known to be hypertensive.

Supplements available: Red Kooga Ginseng (English Grains); Sanatogen Korean Ginseng Capsules

## Royal Jelly

In nature royal jelly is fed exclusively to the queen bee, enabling her alone to become fertile and lead a long and productive life. It provides a rich source of vitamins, minerals and amino acids. It is likely that while it is vital for the queen bee, it has few, if any, benefits for people when studied scientifically. But the queen bee's reliance on it provides some people with a 'fairytale' reason for taking it. They just think it 'does you good', but can't rationalise it to my satisfaction.

Supplements available: Fresh Royal Jelly Capsules (Evans); Golden Health Royal Jelly with Honey; Sanatogen Royal Jelly

# Glossary

**Analgesic**    Painkiller – aspirin, paracetamol, ibuprofen.

**Antibiotic**    A 'naturally' produced substance which destroys or inhibits the growth of germs within the body.

**Anticholinergic**    A chemical that prevents the passage of impulses down 'reflex' nerve pathways in the body and so can relieve symptoms or produce a beneficial effect. The substance hyoscine can do this. It is used in medicines which prevent the bowel cramps associated with irritable bowel syndrome.

**Antihistamine**    A medicine which relieves the symptoms caused by a histaminic response in the tissues. Histamine belongs to a group of chemicals known as the amines. These are released by tissues when they are inflamed and the histamine causes many of the unpleasant symptoms that arise.

**Anti-inflammatory**    A medicine which reduces the swelling, redness, pain and overheating in inflamed tissues of the body. These can be caused by the damage of an accident, an infection or an allergy. A common example is aspirin, which can be given to remove such inflammation – and the associated pain – in an arthritic joint, for example.

**Antipyretic**    A medicine which helps to bring down the body's temperature, which rises when an infection is present. Such a rise in temperature can, in itself, cause feelings of illness. Paracetamol and aspirin are antipyretics.

**Antiseptic**    A chemical substance which prevents sepsis – another name for a harmful infection. In everyday use, the word describes those substances which can be used on or in the body.

**Antispasmodic**     A medicine taken to relieve spasm in muscles (also see anticholinergic).

**Antitussive**     A medicine taken to relieve a cough.

**Astringent**     A substance which dries up excessive secretion – usually by being applied to the surface of the skin or a lining membrane in the throat.

**Decongestant**     A medicine which removes congestion – often water – from inflamed tissues. Nasal drops for a bunged-up nose are an example.

**Emollient**     A substance which softens and soothes.

**Expectorant**     A medicine which 'loosens the phlegm' and allows lung secretions to be coughed up more readily.

**Keratolytic**     An application which dissolves the top, hard, non-living layers of the skin, which are made of keratin. This can make it easier for effective medicines to penetrate into the deeper, living layers of the skin.

**Linctus**     Syrupy liquid containing a variety of ingredients, all of which are given to soothe or loosen the cough.

**Pessary**     A medicated, usually bullet-shaped object, designed to dissolve in and deposit medicines within the vagina.

**Prostaglandin**     A naturally occurring chemical, widely spread throughout the body and in many different forms. The prostaglandins play a part in regulating blood pressure or body temperature; the way in which the blood clots; the acid secretion within the stomach; and in the control of inflammation – to mention only a few.

**Seborrhoeic**     Associated with excessive secretion of sebum produced by sebaceous glands at the bottom of hair follicles.

**Suppository**     A bullet-shaped object designed to dissolve and deliver medicines in the lower bowel.

**Vasoconstrictor**     A substance which constricts the tiny arteries – the arterioles – and can prevent or treat congestion as a result.

# Useful Addresses

**Ainsworth Homoeopathic Pharmacy**, 38 New Cavendish Street, London, W1M 7LH. Telephone: 071 935 5330.

**British Homoeopathic Association**, 27a Devonshire Street, London, W1N 1RJ. Telephone: 071 935 2163

**Homoeopathic Development Foundation**, 1st Floor West, 9 Cavendish Square, London, W1M 9DD. Telephone: 071 629 3205

**National Institute of Medical Herbalists**, 9 Palace Gate, Exeter EX1 1JA. Telephone: 0392 426022 (Mrs Chacksfield)

**Proprietary Association of Great Britain**, Vernon House, Sicilian Avenue, London WC1. Telephone: 071 242 8331 (Can be contacted for information on the non-prescription medicine industry as well as self-medication.)

**Raynaud's and Scleroderma Association Trust**, 112 Crewe Road, Alsager, Cheshire, ST7 2JA. Telephone: 0270 872 776